Carb Cycling Practice and Lifestyle Box Set Bundle

A Painless Diet Plan Based on Metabolic Science Made Easy for Men and Women

John Carver

Carb Cycling

The Science and Practice of Mastering Your Metabolism

John Carver

Table of Contents

Introduction

I want to thank you for purchasing this book *"Carb Cycling – The Science and Practice of Mastering Your Metabolism"* and hope that this book helps you grasp the idea of the carb cycling diet better and accomplish your fitness goals.

Are you someone who is struggling to live a healthy life in a market of unhealthy products? Are you tired of not being able to follow diet plans that help you progress? Is your wish to lose weight in a healthy manner? If the answer to all of these questions is yes, your search has come to an end!

This book will tell you how you can achieve all your fitness goals by following a fun diet plan, which will keep you both interested and healthy at the same time! You'll be surprised how many of your favorite foods you won't have to sacrifice.

Many myths around dieting need to be busted, especially those that suggest starvation as an option. Another misconception is that exercise alone can help you achieve your fitness goals. There is an undue erasure of the role nutrient consumption plays in body transformation. This book will help you understand precisely how.

Carb cycling is the answer to all your worries because it balances the comfort of fun food consumption with customized exercise plans! If you are a bodybuilder, trainer, athlete or someone merely looking to live a healthy life, you must pay attention to the flexible diet that carb cycling is. It can be customized to suit your needs.

The best part is that its strategies are affordable and won't end up burning a hole in your pocket.

The carb cycling diet is the answer to all your worries. It won't only help you lose those extra pounds but also help you get in touch with the healthy lifestyle we all need to survive.

Most diet plans have unhealthy side effects, but carb cycling is entirely safe and does not pose a risk to your body's functioning.

To get pointers and dos and don'ts on how exactly you should go about this carb cycling journey, you need to check out this book. It has information ranging from the science behind carb cycling to how exactly you can practice it at home safely. You can find particular guidelines on how you can get your carb cycling coach through online applications and have full control over the redefinition of your fitness journey.

So what are you waiting for? Read through the pages of this book to uncover multiple secrets about your dream diet.

Chapter One:
What is Carb Cycling?

Fitness is often directly contingent on the nature of nutrient consumption a person engages in daily. The concept of carb cycling is based on the regulation of the intake of carbohydrates to achieve health and fitness goals. The process requires the understanding of the unique requirements of each and implementing a customized diet, which is appropriate for a person's body type.

This approach can help you achieve your health goals by bringing about transformations in the macronutrient consumption schedule.

For it to be implemented, thorough information about your body is required, such as a proper understanding of your medical history. This information is combined with the necessary strategies included in the approach of carb cycling.

To better understand the idea of carbohydrate cycling, you need to be well-versed with the fine details of the program. A good starting point is to understand the meaning of carbohydrates and their function. They are a type of macronutrient that each body needs for energy generation and to fulfill some vital features. These nutrients are derived from the consumption of food substances as the body doesn't manufacture carbohydrates for itself. The primary function of carbohydrates is to provide quick energy generation within the body.

They are made by components such as starch and sugar found in food items such as rice.

Apart from the swift production of energy, these substances are transformed into glycogen upon reaching the liver. The most important role of carbohydrates is to provide fuel for high-intensity activities. The energy required for such events need to be produced in swift intervals, and the body fuels this need by burning carbohydrates.

Simply defined, carb cycling is the approach whereby your diet is structured around the method of increasing and decreasing carbohydrate consumption through a specific period. This could be a weekly or a monthly plan depending on your requirements. It is beneficial for achieving weight loss goals. An individual needs to consume the required amount of carbohydrates to remain fit. A deficiency or excess of carbohydrates can result in an imbalance within the body, resulting in weight loss or gain.

There is a common belief that exercising is the ultimate way to shed extra fat. However, strategies such as carb cycling prove that regular consumption of nutrients can play an important scientific role in the rejuvenation of the body. This method of regulating carbohydrates in diets was initially used by professionals such as bodybuilders and those involved in athletic activities. However, in recent times, the method has become a popular strategy for fitness enthusiasts in maintaining their health.

To further explain the simplicity of carb cycling, one must understand the necessary steps involved in following this diet plan. It is a culmination of high carbohydrate consumption days and low carbohydrate consumption days. The choice of these days is based on the intensity of physical activity a person participates in for any given 24-hours.

The intake of protein and fat remain almost constant on each day. On days when an individual has to indulge in rigorous training, the carbohydrate intake has to be high enough to meet the energy demands of the body. Therefore, the consumption is relatively more than other days. On days when an individual is at rest, the carbohydrate intake has to be lower than the workout day as the body does not require the extra carbohydrate consumption.

Carb cycling is based on a strategy of manipulating carbohydrate consumption to control the body's fat generation process. It is achieved by fluctuating intake of carbohydrates if and when required. The concept of body-hacking comes into play to see relevant results through the diet. This hacking is based on a thorough and intimate knowledge of one's specific body type.

The common problem for dieters is that they gain back the lost weight not long after they stop dieting. It is, therefore, essential to maintain a proper routine involving a perfect mix of exercise and carb cycling to see effective results.

Body Knowledge

There are multiple dieting strategies available separate from carb cycling such as ketogenic diets. However, carb cycling has some unique health benefits that set it apart from other approaches. This is so that it suits the needs of specific body types. However, to uncover these benefits, one must understand the details for their body type.

The human body, male or female, can be separated according to three types; "Ectomorph," "Mesomorph," and "Endomorph."

An individual's body structure is not merely based on how physicality can be analyzed visually. It also tells us about the differing inner responses the body has to nutrient consumption. This is based on recording effects on an individual's hormones and nervous system. Each individual

11

has a distinct metabolism. Therefore, regulating the consumption of nutrients for each body type can have remarkable results. For this, the identification of body type is extremely important.

Among the categories mentioned above, no one individual can completely identify with a specific body type. However, the differentiation assists the individual in getting a basic idea of how they must regulate their diet to achieve the most effective results. Exercising, weight training, yoga, or any other physical activity of choice is still important in achieving health goals holistically. Every person responds to nutrient intake and regulation of carbohydrates differently, exercising enhances the ability of the diet to produce results enormously. Carbohydrate consumption is better in scenarios when the body is actively utilizing the nutrients it receives.

The effects produced by strategies of carb cycling are contingent on specific body requirements. Therefore, the plan should be customized according to the person's physical structure. Due to this, it is very important to grasp the specifications of the three body types to come up with strategies to influence changes in physicality.

Ectomorphs

People who belong in this category are petite, lean, and possess smaller joints than others. Generally, such people are tall and skinny with lean muscle and long, thin limbs. Their muscles are generally tender. However, they possess an extremely swift metabolism, which makes them less susceptible to any weight gain.

Individuals belonging to this category are very unlikely to put on weight; therefore, it is easier for them to indulge in activities such as overeating without gaining much fat. The only way they can gain weight is when they are consuming large amounts of calories. Therefore, with average calorie consumption, they need to engage in workouts that aren't very long but are intense in nature. There should be a special focus on nurturing muscle formation. One nutrient that is important for them is protein, and this can be consumed through special supplements. Since they can shed fat without much struggle, there shouldn't be too many problems involved in harboring lean muscle.

Mesomorphs

This body type is perfect for bodybuilding. Bodies belonging to this category are generally athletic with a bone structure that is medium in frame and size. These bodies can harbor muscle gain because they possess strong growth hormones and the masculine hormone testosterone. Body fat is in check due to higher muscle mass.

Individuals belonging to this category are more susceptible to gain fat; therefore, they must keep the number of calories they consume in check. Their exercises must include some heavy weight lifting coupled with cardio exercises to mitigate the tendency of fat accumulation.

Endomorphs

People belonging to this category often possess shorter builds that are more susceptible to fat accumulation. They have thick arms and legs, which may often put them into the category of being overweight. However, this is just a generalized assumption that does not take into account how their bodies are naturally susceptible to gaining fat. They have strong muscles, yet they often appear to have soft features due to the higher mass of fat they possess. Since they have a higher capacity to consume insulin, their tolerance for carbohydrates is much lesser.

Therefore, the ability to store energy is also higher within this body type.

Their metabolism is not as fast as their other counterparts. People belonging to this category need to constantly do some physical activity to maintain healthy fat formation and prevent unnecessary weight gain. For instance, when people with this body type engage in carb cycling, the intake of carbohydrates will probably be regulated to be lesser than usual since its accumulation coupled with sporadic physical activity results in weight gain.

Once the individual has a basic idea of which of the three categories they identify their bodies with, the next step would be to identify the specific ways the body can be 'hacked' to produce desirable results using carb cycling.

Body Hacking

Body hacking is the next step in determining the nature of the carb cycle that an individual can use to bring positive changes to their body. In this stage, the individual experiments with various diets and strategies to determine what exactly suits their body. Although bodies can be categorized roughly, each genetic makeup is unique and it is pertinent to determine a customized carbohydrate intake pattern.

This process is initiated after one has a general idea about the baseline of the carb cycling pattern. It involves working with different methods of food consumption and exercise to identify the combination that is most appropriate for them.

It can be placed under the category of 'biohacking.' This procedure was initially used by scientists and other curious individuals solely for experimental purposes. In recent times, the strategies of this process have been utilized by individuals all over the globe to heal their physical problems. It instills a sense of balance and positivity for the benefit of their mental health. It is used to increase stamina and performance, and can often prove to be beneficial for overall fitness.

The way to practice biohacking is to cut out unhealthy food consumption. The only way carb cycling can be effective is when the body is supplied with no unnecessary fats, proteins and carbohydrates, for instance, fast foods. Sometimes people consume supplements to lose weight, yet these attempts are often ineffective because nobody accounts for their unhealthy diet habits. Therefore, it is essential to keep in mind that 70 percent of the diet is natural. It should not possess preservatives found in unprocessed foods. Organically prepared ingredients mixed with healthy food intake is the first step to achieve results by using this method.

The base of consumption should be made up of whole foods that contain multiple nutrients required by the body to fulfill its essential functions. These can be discovered in fruits and vegetables. It is recommended to consume more or less six servings of both in a day. Berries help in detoxification of the body, so it is important to consume them with vegetables each day. They contain important fibers that help in intestinal health, along with essential minerals and vitamins.

Another important step in biohacking is to focus on hydration. For instance, the body faces dehydration during sleep. Therefore, it is essential to keep water intake at one or two glasses as soon as you wake up. This not only hydrates the body but also rejuvenates the internal organs to function throughout a hectic day.

Sleep is an important factor for any diet to work. A good six hours of sleep is the least amount of time you should give daily to resting. This rejuvenates the body and opens the mind. This is important because mental health also impacts your body.

Therefore, it must be ensured that the mind is well-rested to initiate the maintenance of good health.

The benefits of biohacking include better body mass composition, prevention of diseases, enhanced cognition, and mental focus. A balanced body mass composition ensures that the fat in your body is not more than the muscle mass.

This ensures a lean and healthy body structure, which is the aim of most dieting techniques. Biohacking strengthens the body's ability to heal. It decreases susceptibility to diseases by eliminating unhealthy practices from daily life. As mentioned earlier, a person's mental capacity influences the ability of their body to function appropriately. Through biohacking techniques, such as carb cycling, the mind receives the care needed for recovery.

Body Reprogramming

The nature of carb cycling is more advanced than other diet plans. To get your body adjusted to this diet plan, it is essential to create proper routines. They guide not only food intake but also physical activity. This diet is based on the regulation of carbohydrates according to the energy requirement of the body. There has to be proper separation of low carbohydrate days and high carbohydrate days.

Low carbohydrate days are generally those that don't require indulgence in a lot of physical activity. Therefore, the requirement for energy generation is also less than other days. There could be either two or three low carbohydrate days in a week to create a balance between low carbohydrate days and high carbohydrate days

High carbohydrate days include training and workout days. The body goes through rigorous physical activity on these days, requiring a large amount of energy supply to sustain its functioning. The carb cycling method reprograms the body by feeding it with only the perfect amount of carbohydrates to meet the demand for sufficient energy generation.

The process of body reprogramming begins with the identification of the set goals the individual wants the body to achieve. This can be achieved by being considerate of multiple factors—for instance, body composition goals that deal with weight loss. Therefore, carbohydrate intake is regulated to achieve those specific results.

To present a picture of what a general carb cycling week would look like, imagine a mixture of two high carb days, two moderate carb days and three low carb days. However, there are differences in carb cycling experiences and patterns that are customized according to body requirements. For instance, the carb intake of an athlete or bodybuilder on a training day will be much higher than that of a person trying to lose a few pounds. This is due to the different responses each way of body programming produces.

In carb cycling, the body is reprogrammed to adhere to a fixed weekly routine with properly drawn out menus and timings for each day to achieve the desired goal. Its complexity arises from sustaining such a regimented lifestyle. It needs to take into account the amount of fat and protein consumption, exercising habits, and body type.

Chapter Two:
Cycling Theory

The most daunting aspect of dieting for weight loss is the 'weight loss plateau' that you hit after a few weeks of being on a diet plan. Once the body gets used to your standard diet and calorie intake, it will impede the burning of fat. Slower metabolism equals slower weight loss. Getting past a weight loss plateau is one of the greatest challenges that require a scientific approach to diet and exercise. Carb cycling, which has its roots in the reality of bodybuilders, has now become a popular dieting method for anyone who wants to burn fat while retaining lean muscle. Several concepts of nutrition that were erstwhile practiced only by elite sports persons have similarly become widely practiced. Counting the macronutrients in your diet, dieting for body re-composition and re-feeding days are used as quick boosts to attain a fitness goal.

Carb cycling, following this trend, has entered the mainstream. It involves 'cycling' between some days of high carbohydrate consumption and some days of low carbohydrate consumption. Healthy high carb foods include quinoa, oats, bananas, vegetables and protein, buckwheat, sweet potatoes, beetroots, and oranges, etc. Low carb foods like nuts, fish, eggs, oils, leafy vegetables, apples, blueberries, and strawberries, etc. are healthy fats and keep the appetite satiated as well.

While many people perform this 'cycle' alternating every month or week, the most effective way to get weight loss results from this method is to alternate one or two days between your low carb and high carb meal plans. Various factors may affect the program of carb intake designed for the individual:

- Body Composition Target: Some individuals, such as athletes, prefer a low intake of carbs during a diet and a high intake during a performance phase.

- Training: Carb intake can be suited to fit the intensity of the training the individual is participating in.

- Body Fat Levels: The lower the body fat percentage, the greater the number of high carb blocks.

- Refeeding Days: One or more than one day of a very high carb consumption act as refeeding days during a long diet.

Maintaining a calorie deficit and not allowing your metabolism to plateau as you coordinate intake with exercise optimizes performance to achieve lean body mass. If the body receives a limited amount of carbs, it uses fat as the primary source of energy resulting in body fat loss. While not regulating carb intake, the body's preferred energy source is carbohydrates. Hence, strategically approaching carb intake can power up the impact of workouts. Fitness today does not merely entail a low body mass; it also entails physical strength, endurance, energy levels, and a healthy diet. All these components are combined in the carb cycling diet, and if carried out properly can have the desired twin result of fat loss with muscle gain.

High Loading, Low Loading, and Calories

It is a common fitness myth that carbs slow down weight loss. The confusion surrounding carbs is caused by restrictive diets or fad diets. They lead to the general belief that it is healthy to eliminate carbs from the diet. They are necessary for healthy bodily functions. However, if the right carbs are consumed from the right sources in proper amounts, they can help burn fat. Eliminating carbs from your diet can slow down metabolism and prevent weight loss. So how does this diet method work?

While there are no formal scientific definitions of 'carb cycling,' there are a few general understandings of it. While working under a constant daily calorie limit, carb limits are fluctuated depending on the day.

A 'low carb' block would require consuming fifty grams or fewer of carbohydrates in a day. The other macronutrients in the diet such as proteins and fats would need to fulfill the calorie limit, and the diet is adjusted accordingly. Non-starchy and leafy veggies, and nuts, etc. are recommended.

A 'high carb' block would demand consuming half of your total calorie limit from carbs. The proportion of other macronutrients would fall but within healthy limits. Some high carb veggies are potatoes, corn, and legumes. One may avoid gluten and dairy as well. However, carbs must not come from processed foods, preservatives, added sugars or alcohol.

As we can see, the foods consumed on both carb blocks are not different; however, they are consumed in different quantities that make a world of difference for achieving smaller weight targets. They seem impossible to achieve otherwise. An average carb-cycling plan could include eating high carbs on Monday and Wednesday and eating low carbs on Tuesday, Thursday, and Friday. All calorie intake comes from healthy alternatives to the average diet. Results are best achieved when this diet plan is combined with a workout plan to match. Low carb days must be combined with high-intensity interval training and a lot of cardio workouts to tap into the fat reserves of the body and burn it off. High carb days are accompanied with strength training to increase muscle mass and give a leaner look simultaneously.

Many testimonials, as well as studying the effects of carb-rich and a carb deficit diet, reveal the efficiency of this method. There is no one way to practice carb cycling or any wrong way to practice it. You must be attuned to the needs of your body and adjust your workouts if there is fatigue on low carb days. Care must be taken that whichever calorie limit and carb block you follow, your food should be rich in nutrients. It also requires immense self-discipline and adherence and should not be practiced for very long terms.

Glucose versus Fat

A nutrient is any substance that an organism needs to survive and thrive. Widely, there are two types of nutrients. Those required by the organism in smaller quantities such as vitamins and minerals are called micronutrients. Conversely, those required in larger quantities are called macronutrients. Carbohydrates are a macronutrient, along with fat and protein. Complex carbohydrates, which are long-chain molecules of sugar, are digested and broken down into glucose and later converted to glycogen to be stored in fat cells due to the action of insulin. Insulin delivers glucose to the cells of the body whenever they need immediate energy. When the glucose is no longer needed, i.e., when the physical activity ends, the leftover glucose is transformed into glycogen and stored for later.

This is the chemical reaction behind how metabolism is affected by the intake of macronutrients. Getting the appropriate amount of carbs at the right times makes your body produce a balanced amount of hormones. These are hormones like thyroid and leptin. However, having too much carb percentage in your daily intake can stimulate insulin release more than the healthy number and cause fat deposits.

Having successive low carb days makes the body use its stored glycogen and burn fat ketone. High carb days are necessary for re-feeding and maintaining calorie and nutrition equilibrium. This implies that while your body can choose to burn either stored carbs or fat during physical activity, it must be encouraged to shift toward the latter simply because it is easier to burn carbohydrates. It must be trained in that direction.

Burning fat for fuel also has many other benefits (which is also called ketosis). It reduces cravings for sugar, improves concentration, balances cholesterol and blood glucose levels, and gives clearer skin. To use up the glycogen stored in muscles and organs such as the liver, a low carb diet is essential.

Glycogen stored in the body is used when the body is not getting energy from food intake. In what is called 'Glycogenolysis,' a compound called glucagon converts the glycogen stored in the liver back to glucose and takes it into the bloodstream. This is how energy is provided to the body until the next food intake. If carbohydrates are consumed continuously, the body will always prioritize burning glucose and store the excess as body fat. If the carbohydrates consumed are more than can be stored as glycogen (the upper limit is 600 mg), then it has to be stored inside fat cells. In this way, consistent overeating and intake of carbs can cause gradual weight gain.

To shift from glycogen to fat, the body must be restricted from getting access to glucose and glycogen. Burning fat instead of glycogen also keep one energized and prevents fatigue. On high carb days, which are to be accompanied by high-intensity workouts, you can prevent the depletion of energy stored in body cells. The human body is programmed to protect itself in the case of weight loss by increasing the need to eat, storing a greater percentage of fat in the body, and slowing down metabolism.

Manipulating your diet to lower carb intake and to correspond it to certain workouts, helps raise muscle and reduce body fat. In the longer run, it also manipulates the whole body into making the choice of burning fat over carbs. A regular application of the carb-cycling method can keep the body wired that way. This it is not just a matter of working hard, but working smart with all the specific needs of your body in mind.

Metabolism

The word metabolism has come up frequently in the last few pages. Before we try to understand the impact of carb intake on it, we must first understand what it involves. It is the process by which the body converts what is consumed in the form of food and drink into energy. It is a complex biochemical process by which calories are combined with oxygen. Energy is required by the body at all times, even when it is at rest, for hidden functions such as blood circulation, respiration, and cell repair, etc. Metabolism or basal metabolic rate can be defined as the rate at which calories are used to provide energy to the body. It is not only genetic but influenced by a lot of factors such as body size, composition, sex, and age. External factors like thermogenesis and the amount of exercise you get also changes the metabolic rate.

The digestive processes that converts carbs into energy are outlined in the previous section. Even beyond weight loss in numbers, carb cycling improves metabolism consistently and for the long-run. There are various motives for this. It helps to not only gain muscle but also to retain it because it encourages protein synthesis. If fat is burned on low carb days, muscle is gained on high carb, intense workout days. This simultaneous action is necessary not just for fitness but also for the overall health of the body. The sensitivity of the body to insulin is also impacted when there is improper carb intake, too many carbs, and your body becomes resistant to insulin. A diet low in carbs or one whereby glycogen is not being continuously stored naturally corrects this desensitization. It prevents type 2 diabetes and other insulin-related diseases.

Through carb-cycling, the whole body can be tricked into opting for a certain set of healthier choices than it is bound to. The biggest of them is the choice to make fats and not carbohydrates, which is its favorite fuel source. The more stored fat cells are used up, the likelier you are to enter a state of ketosis and burn fat from every place in the body.

Carb-cycling is also a sustainable diet approach. It tries to create a balance through fluctuation as opposed to persistently repeating the same calorie deficit. It allows the body to adapt to it by slowing down its metabolism. Consistently regulating carbs not only keeps weight loss consistent, but it also improves physical performance. It is popular among athletes and bodybuilders. This fluctuation opens a pathway for a bigger variety of foods to be included in the diet and hinders stress and boredom generated by a monotonous diet. The variety also makes sure that dieting doesn't have to be accompanied by the feeling of being hungry at all times as a healthy carb-rich diet makes you feel full for a longer time.

If a low carb diet is maintained for a very long period, it decreases the intake of thyroids and reduces the basal metabolic rate. Carb cycling encourages thyroid hormone levels, which regulate the basal metabolic rate, therefore allowing the body to lose fat. Enough carbs in the body also maintain physical performance by preventing muscle wear and tear. High carb days also work on a self-sustaining basis, that is, if low carb days increase the metabolism of the body then the high carb day does not set back weight loss since it is only a cheat day and not a consistent consumption of carb-rich foods that can be stored in the cells of the body. These cheat days keep the mind and body nourished and invested in the diet.

Carbs are also a healthier energy source than is commonly believed; if one cuts out refined sugar, processed foods, etc. it gradually breaks down muscle to make it stronger and repairing muscles requires energy, which is supplied through carbs. By restricting the intake of junk food, cycling also regulates and balances hormone levels, including testosterone and estrogen. Low carbs in your diet enhance the function of the mitochondria, so it uses energy from body cells more efficiently.

High carb intake allows you to exercise for longer periods of time and improve strength and endurance. The overall impact of carb cycling on digestive health and the health of the gut cannot be undermined. Carbs encourage mucus release and prevent acid corrosion of the gut lining. As a lifestyle change, carb cycling also pushes you to opt for healthier plant-based foods as opposed to fatty meats, which also provide the body with fiber and micronutrients.

Carb cycling, while it requires sufficient attention and self-discipline, can be adapted to any kind of lifestyle, whether that of an athlete or a commoner. It combines the innovative components of modern-day fitness tools like intermittent fasting, ketosis, and healthy eating to prolong the results achieved from traditional diet and exercise modules of fitness. It also focuses on a well-rounded increase in the ability of a body to make healthy decisions for itself in the long-run. It gets rid of the psychological disillusionment you feel when consistent diet and exercise do not yield any visible results. It contributes to both the body and the mind.

Chapter Three:
Metabolism

Simply defined, metabolism is the term used for referring to the chemical reactions in the body that take place in the cells of organisms. This process is what furthers the sustenance of life, through enabling growth as well as reproduction in the body. Organisms sustain the structures of their bodies in the ecosystem through this process. Processes such as digestion, chemical reactions that transmit nutrients from one cell to another, are possible because of your metabolism. This is called intermediary metabolism.

There are two types of metabolism, catabolism and anabolism.

The first type, catabolism, is the process where organic matter is broken down to be absorbed by the body. The second type, anabolism, utilizes energy to build cells and construct its components, for instance, nucleic acids and proteins.

There are a series of chemical reactions that take place during the process of metabolism. These are arranged in metabolic pathways that enable the transformation of chemicals from one stage to another through a series of steps. Enzymes are the catalysts for facilitating this chemical reaction. Any chemical reaction needs a catalyst to trigger it. In this scenario, the activity would not be able to occur without the help of enzymes. This is due to the fact they generate responses to signals in cells and help in the regulation of metabolic pathways. This speed the metabolism operates is named metabolic rate.

The metabolism also acts as a detector of substances. It determines whether the substances are nutritious and useful or fatal and poisonous. Other chemicals are involved in this metabolic process, namely carbohydrates, amino acids, proteins, nucleotides, coenzymes, cofactors and minerals.

Specific to the study of carb cycling is the idea of carbohydrate metabolism. It is a biochemical process that occurs in the body to ensure a constant supply of energy for all living cells. The most important carbohydrate for this process is glucose. The process of glycolysis occurs to break down glucose, which makes an entry into the Krebs cycle, where it goes through a process of oxidative phosphorylation to generate adenosine triphosphate (ATP).

During the process of digestion, carbohydrates are broken down into simple and soluble sugar. After this, they are taken through the intestinal wall to the circulatory chamber and taken to different organs of the human body. Carbohydrates begin undergoing the digestion process in the mouth, which consists of saliva and salivary amylase reacting with starches to break them down. The last stage of digestion occurs when monosaccharides are absorbed from the epithelium of the small intestine. This is followed by the process of cellular respiration once the absorbed monosaccharides are transported to different tissues.

Carbohydrate is extremely necessary for metabolic pathways. Their synthesis happens in plants during the process of photosynthesis. The energy that these plants absorb from sunlight is stored during photosynthesis. This is followed by the consumption of plants by animals and fungi. These stored carbs are broken down by these organisms through the process of cellular respiration to provide energy to their cells. There is a temporary storage of the energy released from carbohydrates in the form of high-energy molecules such as

ATP, which are stored for later utilization for different cellular processes.

The consumption of carbohydrates by humans occurs in different forms. However, in all scenarios, complex carbohydrates are systematically broken down into simple monosaccharides through the process of digestion. This is the process that is responsible for the generation of glucose, fructose, and galactose. Among these chemicals, almost 80 percent is glucose. Therefore, it forms the primary structure. It is distributed to cells and tissues of the body where it is further broken down into glycogen or stored. During the process of aerobic respiration in the human body, the release of energy is derived through metabolizing glucose and oxygen. The formation of water and carbon dioxide also occurs. These are considered to be byproducts. While glucose is undergoing this process, fructose and galactose are transported to the liver where they can be transformed into glucose.

There are few simple carbohydrates that consist of enzymatic oxidation pathways, but a very negligible number of complex carbohydrates possess this. For instance, the breaking down of disaccharide lactose to glucose and galactose creates a requirement for lactase to act as a catalyst.

Role of Water for Metabolic Activity

Water serves as an essential bodily fluid in organisms. In the context of metabolic activity, it is indispensable as it plays a central role in the process of digestion, absorption, transportation, and synthesis of fluids. It helps in the detoxification of the body by cleansing internal organs and flushes out toxic waste. All biochemical reactions that occur in the body require some kind of lubricant to facilitate the reaction, and water serves the primary purpose in this regard. It also aids thermoregulation required by the human body to function and acts as a lubricant of different cavities, which include joints.

Contemporary research has led physiologists to discover brand new functions of cellular water since it is the main constituting substance of the cells. Water found in the cells paves the way for passing water among intracellular and extracellular compartments. These are the central factors that affect the volume of cells; this, in turn, regulates a plethora of functions carried out by cellular activity. Examples of such cellular activity include metabolism, which is the driving force of the body. Other examples include epithelial transport, hormone release, excitation, cell proliferation, migration, or the death of a cell.

The human body consists of almost 60 percent water and is important for almost all bodily functions. It is often ignored in literature and mainstream scientific discussion as an important nutrient. The consideration of carbohydrates, proteins, or fats as the sole macronutrients involved in energy generation in the human body is also fallacious. On close consideration of the constant supply of water needed for the body to process energy-producing functions, one realizes that water serves as perhaps the most important micronutrient.

To carry out any diet, it is necessary to regulate nutrient intake. The same applies to water since studies have pointed out certain loopholes in the use of water as a body-hacking mechanism.

This definition of the nutritious content value of water is called hydration status or fluid balance. The reason why the specific nutritional definition of water as a nutrient is a difficult task is because the human body does not include a reserve of water. Due to this, fluids need to be constantly recycled. The ideal way to measure fluid balance is to determine fluid gain and loss, which can be done through nutrition and metabolic water production. The manner it can be traced is through the urinary system, the respiratory tract, the gastrointestinal system and the skin in controlled conditions of the environmental system over a fixed and short amount of time.

Water levels and fluid dynamics tend to vary for a person over a different period of time, such as the fluid dynamics in the day versus that in the night and vice versa. This difference can ever occur over a few hours. Therefore, even though the overall fluid balance is an important factor, hydration status that is the amount of water a body possesses at a given point of time may provide more insights into metabolic activity as compared to fluid balance.

There are a plethora of markers that exist for measuring hydration status, which include plasma osmolality and sodium concentrations that come under hematologic indices. Apart from this, urine osmolality, specific gravity, and urine color are also considered, which fall under urinary indices. Other markers include bioelectrical impedance, cardiovascular function measures such as blood pressure, heart rate, and orthostatic tolerance.

The purpose of these markers is to draw a reasonable estimation of dehydration, which occurs in the case of a deficiency or over-hydration that occurs due to an overload of fluid in the human body. While these are important markers, they can provide a proper estimation of the exact actual water needs a body may have.

Role of Water in Diet Plans

While it is important to know the science behind the interaction of water with the body to further metabolic activity, you need to know how it can bring benefits to your diet plan. For this, we need to explore the key roles in which water helps to solve multiple problems in the body in furthering processes such as weight loss.

Every dietician advises drinking warm, clean water as an essential factor for sustaining a healthy life protected from illnesses. The body's ability to function in the absence of food is much higher as its ability to process metabolic activity in the absence of water. This also increases life expectancy. Water is not only essential in metabolic processes but also in eliminating toxins. We have discussed in the previous section how water aids in digestion. In the context of diets, specifically carb cycling, water aids in weight loss since food is essentially highly regulated.

The importance of drinking water is incomparable when it comes to the idea of weight loss through a diet. This is because it aids in eliminating calories and keeps the body's constant involuntary tendency to eat in check.

It also paves a way within the body system to carry out bodily processes smoothly.

Because it consists of no calories, it acts as a healthy replacement for extra servings at mealtimes, which can often act as barriers in the body's healthy development. The most essential function is the ability of water to flush out harmful substances from the body.

Humans consume an insane amount of toxins daily, which permeates into the food they eat. Drinking water helps to establish a way out for these toxins and also prevents their harmful side effects from taking control of the body.

Since it flushes unwanted materials like wastes from the metabolic system, it takes a position of extreme essentiality when it comes to regulating the fat in metabolism. As a result of this, the effects of diets aiding weight loss are phenomenal.

Certain recommendations posit that women should consume around 91 ounces of water each day, and men should consume 125 ounces per day. This estimation is derived from the culmination of all secondary sources of water, including beverages and foods.

When it comes to the sole consumption of water, 64 ounces are considered a healthy amount to indulge in daily. It must be kept in mind that these are generalized estimations since the body's water content is largely determined by age, diet, exercise, physical activity, climate, and body composition.

A way to illustrate this would be to consider that when a person is exercising, the amount of water that needs to be consumed rises. This is possible in warm weather conditions too. The loss of water in these scenarios increases on an hourly basis. Water, therefore, must be consumed before commencing a workout as well as when it is going on and afterward.

It must be consumed constantly at short intervals even when the body does not feel thirsty since that is a glaring sign of a dehydrated body.

There are four methods that water intake can be elevated.

Maintain a water tracker

This will enable you to set up reminders for getting your constant fill of water. People often have busy schedules, and it can act as a personal guide to aid you in the journey of healthy dieting. A tracker like this is readily available on the internet and can be downloaded on your smartphone through the app store.

Carry a water bottle at all times

This is an important accessory everyone must have in their bags. In social situations, you are often left dehydrated due to work, and the best method to recall to take care of your body is to carry water everywhere. This will prevent dehydration and also increase water daily water intake considerably.

Consume water via food substances

Fresh fruits and vegetables that are juicy and nutritious contain large amounts of fluids that are essential for your diet. Apart from water, you can make meals out of broth and clear soup. This acts as a light meal profuse with fluids. These foods also contain a negligible amount of calories, therefore they do not add unneeded carbs in the diet. Low-fat skimmed milk and yogurt also play the same role and should be incorporated into your carb cycling diet. Fruits with citrus undertones, such as oranges and grapefruit, also aid in refueling water content in the body.

Personalizing Carb Cycling

Carb cycling follows a set formula of dieting. It functions on a baseline that directs the basic strategy of how one must go about it. Yet to achieve appropriate results, all aspects of the diet need to be adjusted according to personal requirements. Every individual's body is unique, therefore every diet needs to be customized according to specific needs. This can be done by trying different approaches to following carb cycling and gradually figuring out which approach works best.

Carb cycling can work in two ways; it can help you burn unwanted fat and also gain healthy weight. The difference between these two results lies in the number of low carb and high carb days in your diet. The lower the number of carbohydrates you consume, the more weight you will lose. If you add low carb days to your plan, your body gets a chance to burn fat. However, when you add high carb days on a weight loss plan, an anabolic environment is created. You will be gaining muscle and holding onto it due to an increase in amino acid intake and protein synthesis while protein breakdown is reduced. This is why there are simultaneous fat loss and muscle gain in this plan.

Carb cycling manipulates where our body gets fuel. The body's preferred form of fuel energy comes from carbohydrates. Carbohydrates allow your muscles to be full of glycogen stores, and it's really easy for your body to convert it into energy.

However, once you have depleted all the carbs and used all your energy, your body has to find another source of energy to run off. That is when your body starts using fats. This is when the body begins tapping into the stored fat cells of your body, utilizing them, and resulting in weight loss. When the body uses fat instead of carbs as its energy source, you start losing weight faster.

We all respond to carbohydrates differently. On a weight loss diet, people typically go months eating at a calorie deficit every day. The problem with this is that long calorie deficit will ultimately lead to drops in metabolic functions to the point where your initial calorie deficit is now your maintenance. This is when weight loss comes to a halt. Avoiding this and being consistent with carb cycling is the key to weight loss and improved athletic performance.

This is essentially why it's extremely important to figure out the purpose of your diet. Benefits are visible according to specific body hacking techniques, and you must follow a proper baseline to achieve your goals.

Carb cycling fits any lifestyle. It puts you in control of your lifestyle as you learn how to shed weight and make better choices. This diet will leave you feeling more energized and better throughout the day. You get to eat the foods you love without having to eliminate them from your diet. It will help you build more muscle and replace extra fat. The carb cycle period will empower you physically and mentally.

Chapter Four:
The Model

What does it mean to 'diet'? You may imagine it to be an eccentric habit of 'health-freaks' who can discipline their body into surviving on powdered proteins and salad. This traditional image of dieting comes from the side effects of severe self-restriction on food intake. These can cause eating disorders or the general inaccessibility of dieting to people who believe that it is a costly venture. Special 'diet foods' were often marketed to a potential health-conscious crowd of consumers. However, with more research on the body and its nutrition needs, the new fitness trend is aimed at a holistic and sustainable training of the body. You can call it a responsive and responsible health consciousness that tries to accommodate the varying needs of varying shapes.

This means that a lot of common myths about dieting have been shattered in the last few decades. Skipping breakfast as a way of losing weight is no longer encouraged and neither is entirely eliminating foods that you enjoy eating from your diet. Another common myth that has been dispelled is that carbs, in totality, are bad for the body because they are fattening. However, it has been discovered that maintaining a calorie deficit with simultaneous exercise is the best way to shed the pounds. It is the calorie intake that matters more than the kind of macronutrient that is being consumed. That is, no carbs are inherently wrong. Most carbohydrate-rich foods also tend to be rich in calories because they are often supplemented with plentiful calorie toppings, sauces, and sides. Some carbs, however, are both fibrous and nutritious and can keep you feeling full as well as help you cut your calories at the same time.

Carb cycling is not equivalent to traditional dieting. It is not absolutely restrictive and does not treat any foods as good or bad. The focus is more on the quantity of food intake, and the time it is consumed. It also does not have any fixed rules that can be universally observed by everyone who tries carb cycling. The kind of meal plan you have is based directly on your basal metabolic rate, your training schedule, and also your likes and dislikes. Any lack of nutrition can always be supplemented by eating healthy foods that are not carbs on low carb days and any fatigue incurred as a result of weight loss can be overcome by eating healthy carbs on high carb days. This dieting approach does not amount to starvation and undernourishment. It is mindful of the needs of the body, the health of organs, the time it takes for fat to burn and muscle to build, the balance of hormones and the psychological importance of a healthy diet. It is an aggressive as well a constructive strategy that combines the benefits of low carb diets and high-intensity training.

One of the critical reasons for the success of carb cycling as a dietary practice has been due to its nontraditional approach and strategic handling of the concept of calorie restriction.

More Than a Diet

To better explain the uniqueness of carb cycling as a dietary method, in this section there will be a comparison of the approach that regular dieting takes as opposed to the one that carb cycling takes to dieting and weight loss.

As humanity evolved, the creation of large-scale manufacturing industries increased the consumption of mass-produced food items. They contained substances that were not dominant in organic diets. These substances, such as refined sugar, salt, and bread, etc. began to fundamentally alter patterns of human eating and how the body adjusted to such changes. Traditional dieting conceptually looks at the body as a simple machine that functions quantitatively.

The idea of health and fitness itself is looked at as transactional--the more you eat, the heavier you get, and the more you exercise, the more muscle you gain. Hence, calorie counting is all the rage, and calorie restriction is the only surefire way to lose pounds. This is the kind of thought that gave rise to bizarre, ineffective, and dangerous diets such as the grapefruit diet, which focused on quick and temporary weight loss through starvation-like conditions. The use of diet pills that would eliminate hunger even at the cost of nutrition, or laxatives, which would induce diarrhea, was normal among those who aspired to fitness.

With the advent of research into the human body and how the modern diet affects the body, including how different individual components of the food interacts with the body and under what circumstances, there was a greater push to create new, nuanced diets. This shift was encouraged by the affluence of the macro nutrition theory, which was already popular among sportspersons. Physiology was seen as a byproduct not only of how much was consumed but indeed what was consumed and in how much quantity. It is evident that diet and health were looked at far more qualitatively than in traditional dieting.

Dieting trends including intermittent fasting, ketogenic diets, research into healthy alternatives to regular food and plant-based diets, etc. are on the rise. Riding this wave of focus on macro nutrition is also the carb cycling approach, which takes calorie counting to the next level.

Let's look at a sample carb cycling meal plan and exercise routine and then analyze the effects on the average human body:

High Carb Block Meal Plan:

- Breakfast: Boiled eggs, lettuce, mushrooms, whole-wheat/grain bread, fruits
- Lunch: Vegetables, side of lean meat, side of sweet potato
- Pre-Workout: Whey protein, oatmeal, and fruits
- Dinner: Brown rice, side of lean meat/fish, kidney beans, vegetables

Low Carb Block Meal Plan:

- Breakfast: Eggs, bacon slices, mixed vegetables
- Lunch: Salmon/Lean fish salad
- Snack: Mixed nuts
- Dinner Steak, avocado, vegetables

High-Carb Days: 1800 calories

- 50 percent carbs
- 25 percent protein
- 25 percent fat

Low-Carb Days: 1400 calories

- 35 percent carbs
- 35 percent protein
- 30 percent fat

In the average week, high carb days include Monday, Thursday and Friday; low carb days include Wednesday, Saturday and Sunday. High carb days are accompanied by intense weight training and low carb days may be accompanied by light aerobics, with the exception of one or two days that will be rest days.

With a certain amount of adjustment time, people report that they find the calorie count to be manageable and did not report any lethargy or feeling of hunger due to the diet. People who tried carb cycling for a short period reported feeling less bloated and more active. People who tried it consistently reported having better workouts and consistent weight loss over a period of time. Along with it, they also experience better digestion, clearer skin, lower workout-associated muscle pains, and feeling lean and toned.

Value

The low carb diet has been quite the craze in the weight loss world for decades. As mentioned earlier, carbs were targeted as the primary source of weight gain by fitness buffs. They continue to be considered strictly off limits when weight loss is the goal. Many dieting approaches restrict the intake of carbs to a bare minimum without any afterthought of how that would affect the body and its functions.

The premise of the low carb, though, in reality, ignores the entire knowledge associated with the positive effects of consuming carbs, which are manifold. Let us take a look at the myths around carbs and disprove them:

Carbs are the primary source of weight gain

It is not false that foods like pizza and bread will cause weight gain if they are consumed too often. However, it is also true those high carb foods that are also rich in nutrients and fiber can achieve the opposite result. What low carb diets ignore is that it is only simple carbs that are fattening, like simple sugars, refined sugars, and so on. It's complex carbs that don't make you gain weight. What is also important is the kind of carbs you consume and the quantity you consume. It's the carbs with too many calories that should be avoided. White bread, pasta, fried food, and refined flour baked goods are devoid of their nutritional value and rapidly elevate blood sugar levels.

However, there are also carbs that are not refined and considered good carbs. Grains, legumes, and lean meat retain their fiber and have a lot of protein. They elevate your blood sugar level gradually and need less insulin. They make you feel full longer.

Only white foods contain carbs

Due to the fact that certain white foods are the primary source of bad carbs, people also tend to assume that all white foods contain bad carbohydrates. However, white foods like potatoes are extremely good for health. Even if they contain a high amount of carbs, they are also very rich minerals and vitamins like vitamin C and potassium. As long as they are consumed in moderation, they will do well to the body. Such similar good high carb white foods are ginger, pears, cauliflowers, and apples.

Fruits are fattening because they contain carbs

When people start listening to mainstream weight loss advice, they often begin to believe that because fruit naturally contain a lot of sugar, they must be entirely avoided if weight loss is desired. However, fruit need to form an essential part of one's diet. They are extremely rich in nutrients, and their sugar is natural fructose, which, unlike refined sugar, does not harm the body. Fruit contains phytonutrients, vitamins, minerals, and, most importantly, fiber. Fresh fruit must be preferred over packaged juice and must be consumed in moderation since fruit contains calories that can throw your macronutrient proportions out of balance since you will meet your calorie limit only by fruit.

Low carb diets

Low carb diets have shown effectiveness only to better insulin sensitivity, but in the long-run, also cause many other ailments. Low carb diets increase the risk of cardiovascular diseases such as heart attacks and strokes. Those who participate in sports also need carbs as fuel. Good carbs also do not cause inflammation or diabetes. They consist of a high fiber content, which improves digestion. They are also low in gluten.

Body Systems

We will now venture into the scientific complexities of carbohydrates as macronutrients to show that they cannot be universally and generally avoided in the name of health and fitness. Carbohydrates are chemically composed of hydrogen and oxygen, and their two basic compounds are ketones and aldehydes. They form polymers when they combine. Polymers act as molecules for long-term food storage. In plants, they are also structured support. They are comprised of starches, sugars, and fibers present in the food that we consume. They are one of the three macronutrients from which the body contains energy; fats and proteins are the other two.

The National Institute of Health has recommended that the daily intake of carbohydrates for the average adult body to be 135 grams, which is obviously subject to variations in health.

The five types of carbohydrates are monosaccharides, disaccharides, polysaccharides, oligosaccharides, and polyols. There are also simple and complex carbohydrates, the simple ones being sugars consisting of one to two molecules. Complex carbs contain long chains of sugars. It is not complex carbs that cause any of the ill effects that carbs are portrayed to cause. It is the simple carbs present in refined sugars, processed foods, and junk foods that cause harm.

Carb intake helps to regulate body weight. Those who have a high carb diet are more likely to shed weight than those who follow a strictly low carb diet. There are multiple reasons for this. First, carbs contain fewer calories than most foods, even fewer than alcohol. Second, the energy density of a high carb diet is lower, and carbs with fiber make you feel full faster and for longer. This prevents overeating or binge eating. They have a considerably low glycemic index and therefore will take time to digest and keep releasing energy.

Third, the body burns carbs for fuel. Excess carbs are stored for future use. If there is a very low amount of carbs, they are turned into fat and stored in the body. Obesity is less likely in the case of high carb diets than high-fat diets, which is why, rather than blaming only carbohydrates for a spike in obesity, it is more effective to look at the comprehensive lifestyle changes that have caused it. It is the constant rejection of carbs that leads to many lifestyle fads that do not really cause any actual change in the root cause of obesity as we have explained it.

While carbs are often blamed for causing the rise in obesity, there are a lot of unrelated reasons that contribute to obesity. These include very little physical activity from a sedentary lifestyle, a flawed sleep cycle which affects the body functions, the heavy consumption of junk food regularly, the consumption of processed foods that contain additives, colorings and sugars, and the stress that you might be under that can alter your eating habits. As the standards and habits of living change, more and more causes for obesity can be identified.

Diabetes is also far more widespread than it was two decades ago. It is a metabolic disorder that does not allow the body to regulate its glucose levels well. Insulin sensitivity is directly linked to blood glucose regulation. It is not proven that sugar consumption directly causes type 2 diabetes, but it is linked to obesity. This is an effect of refined sugar consumption.

The mouth contains different enzymes and bacteria that act upon carbs when they are chewed and breaks them down. It leads to the production of acid, which affects the tooth enamel. This is neutralized by the saliva present in the mouth. Saliva also rebuilds enamel. Sugar is a fermentable carb. If it is consumed too often, the natural saliva enamel repair system is thrown out of balance.

Carbs drastically improve physical performance because they provide fuel for muscles and maintain glycogen stores during and after a workout. Beta-glucans regulate the body cholesterol levels; fiber improves fecal health, blood glucose can be regulated, lactulose speeds up intestinal transit and plaque in the teeth can be reduced by consuming xylitol.

It has been discussed that the cycling approach has many health benefits reaching beyond the scope of simple weight loss. Through the above examples, you may realize that instead of focusing on short-term weight reduction, it prepares the body to become a machine of high functionality and better metabolism, which also discourages the gaining of weight once the diet stops. Once the hormone regulation balance in the body has been restored, and the insulin sensitivity has been regulated, it is easier to continue the cycle of diet and exercise because you are not haunted by any health complications, neither are you focused only on dropping pounds. The carb cycling approach will make you accept health and diet-related awareness as a lifestyle choice.

Chapter Five:
Implementation of Carb Cycling

Now that we have explained to you the model and the scientific logic behind the carb cycling dietary approach, let us discuss the implementation of it. After all, a large part of the success of this diet lies in how well it is planned and carried out by you.

This approach requires almost constant monitoring and watchfulness, and should not be analyzed on theoretical value alone. While we cannot generate one standard idea of what implementation of carb cycling will look like, we can try to understand the basic principles of its implementation.

The implementation is done in three parts. First, there is the diet itself. Many individuals, especially non-athletes, often practice their diets alongside their regular routines and that could comprise jobs, families, and other commitments. The division of the high carb and low carb blocs must be done in a way that low carb days coincide with those days on which there is less vigorous activities to be done.

Similarly, high carb days can be reserved for days that demand high energy. The constituent meals of your meal plan should also be filled with produce that is locally grown, fresh, and easy to source. A diet that comprises exclusively of expensive diet foods is not sustainable and could contain many unhealthy preservatives.

The second part is the cycle. This cycle may be mapped out between one high carb day to the other and so on. Mastering the balance between consumption and expenditure of calories is crucial in maintaining a healthy cycle of energy intake and usage. How you transition from a low carb day to a high carb one is also important. The body must be eased into eating more carbs on certain days so that they are given ample time to digest and enter the energy stores of the body. Similarly, complete starvation during low carb days must be avoided by breaking down your food intake into five or six smaller meals and keeping yourself nourished all day. The cycle must also have time to assimilate into your routine and to become a natural part of it.

The third important part of the implementation is the plan. The plan is the careful mixture of diet and exercise that has been planned out to the last detail of when to eat what, and in what quantities. The plan must include accessible and effective ways of working out that are not so tedious you become discouraged from completely utilizing your high carb day energy.

The biggest trick to understanding dieting is that it should not feel disruptive. The body has a way of making the mind reject what does not feel natural to it. When the emotional aspect of eating food was discussed earlier, it was mentioned that disillusionment with your diet is one of the major reasons why you might not successfully carry it out.

The implementation of it must make an effort to make it feel as natural as possible by easing your body into it and taking care of it through the course of the diet. As your carb cycling routine becomes more and more natural to you, you will experience a gain in the benefits you derive from it.

Carb cycling is a way of demanding peak physical performance from the body. The more natural it becomes to you, the closer you are to maximizing your physiological potential.

It might seem contradictory to say that the diet must at once be monitored and natural. The simple solution is that the suggestion of carb cycling is not that monitoring must be done self-consciously. It must be done so that it becomes normal for you to be aware of what you put in your body. This monitoring should be as an important yet mindless element, such as preparing meals.

Two Diets

The idea of monitoring a diet that is based on constant changes might seem rather futile. There are ways, however, by which the monitored data can be used to improve the effectiveness of the diet. If both the low carb and high carb diets are approached as two different diets, then by monitoring their individual effectiveness, we can generate a fuller idea of the cycle. Planning the diet is a game of conjecture—since one never really knows how some diet-exercise combinations will act upon your body. Monitoring it, however, is a fairly scientific and empirical exercise.

Based on the two intersecting aspects of the plan, the diet and the exertion, there are four possible variations of the combinations of days that are created. All these combinations results in days that need a specific kind of meal plan and a specific kind of exercise plan to maximize their potential.

The first is the high-extended exertion day. This is a high carb day that will allow you the time to perform a longer workout that will focus not only on weight but also on strength and endurance. On this day, the meals you plan must be those that take time to digest, so that they will keep releasing energy into the body. Consider whole grains and yogurt combined with high-intensity aerobics for a longer than normal period of time. This is the toughest day you will have during your cycle.

The second is the low extended exertion day. This is the low carb day that comes after another low carb day when the body might suffer a paucity of energy, and the meals you eat on this day must make you feel full even if it is consumed in smaller amounts. Meals can be reared with sweet potatoes and eggs.

Combine this with stretching and light yoga for workout without over exertion.

The third day is the high-burst exertion day. This is the day of refueling and re-feeding. It is the day you consume the maximum carbs and also perform the most intense workouts. You will be combining weight training with cardio workouts. The meals on this day must be loaded with energy and fiber. Bananas, fish and brown rice are good sources of fiber. Hydration is crucial so be sure to drink enough to prevent dehydration.

The fourth day is the low-burst exertion day. This is the low carb day that comes immediately after the refueling day when the energy from eating a lot of carbs the previous day is still left in the body. On this day, you might perform some rigorous yet light aerobics or maybe do a shorter version of your high carb workout. The goal is to lengthen the improved physical performance for as long as possible and to burn as much fat as possible.

Each of these must be evaluated separately because they all have very separate roles in your main diet. As is evident, every meal plays a unique role in the creation of energy for your workout. There are two simultaneous high carb and low carb diets working under the same calorie restriction. Both of the diets need their own set of parameters and their own observations. There will be many foods that will be common for both diets, and a good inventory of what are appropriate serving sizes should be created for the two parallel diets.

The Cycle

Carb cycling can be done in three modes: high load, moderate load, and low load. Each of these three levels have their own corresponding needs and outcomes. They also have their specific intake attached to them. The changes in intake must be consistent with the proportion specified by the carb cycling principle—on high carb days half your calories must come from healthy carbs, and on low carb days nearly 25 percent of your day's calorie intake should be from carbs. The load, or the amount of calories you eat in one day, must be determined by your existing body mass, your body goals and your metabolism rate.

A high-loading carb cycle is appropriate for people who are required to exert themselves physically to a greater degree than the average person. These include professional athletes and also people who play sports or are involved in strenuous jobs such as construction work. The opposite ends of their meal cycle, which is high carb loading and low carb loading, should have a large difference between them.

Since the daily calorie intake of such people is from 4000 to 6000 calories, it is not very difficult to maintain the difference. Their meals also tend to gravitate toward the heavier side, especially before matches. This gives them the requisite energy to overexert themselves for a few hours. On non-match days, they still need high-energy meals because they need to practice and maintain their fitness. Lack of nutrition for such people can lead to muscle cramps and poor performance on the field. A high loading cycle suits them best because it ensures that nutrition is not looked over when trying to become fit.

A moderate loading carb cycle is best for people who have already had a period of training and dieting before they embark on carb cycling. While they might not be professional athletes, they do have a rigorous workout routine and are accustomed to eating healthy. For such people, a moderate carb load that is filled with commonly available food is apt. Since their basal metabolic rate is already high, it is easier for these individuals to digest the food they eat and burn it easily during workouts. However, their bodies still need to be trained to burn far over burning carbs. It's important they carry out the cycle to tune their body to their needs. They can also include different types of exercises in their routine so that they can start gaining muscle.

A low loading carb cycle is the best way for beginners to ease themselves into the world of dieting. The low loading cycle is filled with meals that are simple, easy to prepare, and fulfilling rather than instant energy-giving. A lot of fibrous foods are the best to start with. Since these people are not entirely used to having a rigorous workout routine, their meal plans must be complemented with light stretching, aerobics, yoga and jogging.

The Plan

The carb cycling 'plan' is a long-term commitment to a dieting logic and a certain lifestyle. Apart from the implementation aspects of the diet, there are a few other factors that must be taken care of when you are practicing the diet. The fuel you choose, the methods of monitoring you prefer, the kind of activity you participate in—all form part of the universe in which carb cycling is supposed to function. To make sense of the dieting elements mentioned above, you will have to make them compatible with your schedule. Otherwise, this easy balance will forever be impossible for you.

When divided under these three aspects, the plan is easy to decipher. The first part is the activity. This is addressed to the total exercise and the kind of exercise you prefer on certain days. Some people are satisfied with high-intensity interval training workouts during their high carb days because with an increased physical performance they can take shorter rest breaks and give their best during their session. However, there are those who want to add an extra dimension to their workout by also devoting time to weight training. Weight training has been shown to complement carb cycling well because more fats are burned and more muscle is built. However, exercise is not just limited to high carb days but must also be done during your low carb ones.

Here, too, there are differing opinions as to which is the best workout for the light intake days. There seems to be a special preference for light aerobics since it works out the whole body without unnecessary stress and is quite fun to do. Speed walking, light jogging, yoga, and playing a light sport are all good ways to work out without getting fatigued on low intake days.

The second part is the fuel. These are the few stock good carbs that you will choose to form the base of your diet, the consumption of which will be mostly during high carb days. You should choose a fuel not just from the options available on the internet or only based on its nutritional value in numbers. You should also focus on how the food makes your body feel and whether it does satisfy you and keep you energetic for long.

Your refueling days should also be clearly demarcated, and the meal plans for these days must be very carefully thought out because it is on refueling days that people tend to give themselves a free pass and eat anything they crave. The consumption of a high-fat diet will drain you of energy, and sugar will have the same effect. This is not the result you want at all because a refueling day is so use to leave you with enough energy to power through your cycle. If it is used only as a cheat day its value is seriously compromised.

The third part is monitoring. One of the ways monitoring is made easy on diets for people is if they give the charge of monitoring to someone that they trust. This decreases the amount of work you need to do and also makes sure that you receive an objective view of your health statistics from a neutral party. To make certain the monitoring is efficient you must have a list of all the things you need to periodically measure and a corresponding list of sources where you can measure them. Simple things like weight, size and even blood sugar can be checked at home with the right equipment, but cholesterol levels and hormonal health has to be checked by a professional.

The biggest factor that will command your time is your schedule. To divide the above factors adequately in the free time that you have, you might have to give up on some things such as using your mobile phone too much or sleeping very late.

The point of such any rigorous diet is that you should not have spare time to waste and to make sure that you sleep soundly at night. Other than that, carb cycling does not demand extra workout time, but all the free time that you have between busy days can be devoted to planning your meals and monitoring your body stats. As was mentioned in the introduction to this section, it is imperative that the diet feel as natural as possible, and it must be made to be integrated with your schedule, not stand apart from it. Going to work and going to the gym should carry the same weight in your mind.

Chapter Six:
Good Sources of Carbohydrates

The purpose of this section is to identify healthy sources of carbohydrates that you must incorporate into your diet on your carb recycling journey. A sound understanding of unhealthy carbohydrate foods that must be excluded from your diet is important to ensure the effectiveness of your body-hacking strategy.

In recent years, carbohydrates have garnered a lot of controversies. This is a result of the common belief that carbohydrates cause diabetes and obesity when taken in high amounts. All things considered, nutritionists suggest that you must consume at least half your calories through carbs alone.

The question then becomes, how does one identify healthy sources of carbohydrate intake?

The purpose of this book is to show the right sources and strategies of making your carb cycling journey worthwhile. It has been made clear why carbohydrates are extremely essential macronutrients in your diet. The way to derive these benefits is to consume the right sources of carbohydrates and cut down any carbs that can be harmful.

Through this chapter, you can differentiate between good and carbs to suit your purposes.

This discussion will be divided into three separate sections that will delineate the exact ways you can differentiate between different types of food to ensure they aren't harmful to your diet.

Unprocessed and Unrefined Carbohydrates

Whole grains are important in this section. These can be differentiated on multiple levels, but one of the common determinants is to trace the difference between what packaged graphics represent and the ingredients that are present in them.

Unprocessed carbohydrates are categorized by whole carbohydrates that retain their natural fiber. In the case of refined carbohydrates, the natural fiber erodes due to the processing they undergo. Unrefined carbohydrates are considered as good as they come under the category of whole carbohydrates. Refined carbohydrates, on the other hand, cause a multiplicity of issues that hinder the success of the diet plan.

Some examples of whole carbohydrates are vegetables and whole fruits, whole grains, legumes, and so on. These options are healthy ones to incorporate into your diet.

Some examples of refined carbohydrates are white rice, white pasta, white bread, sweetened juices, and other beverages. These are often the culprits of weight gain when consumed consistently even if not in extremely copious amounts.

The importance of good carbs is irreplaceable when it comes to the process of carb cycling. To accrue the benefits from your intensive diet plan, the consumption of the right kind of carbohydrates is extremely important. They consist of multiple benefits such as lowering cholesterol, regulating blood pressure, and also reducing it in cases of fluctuating or high blood pressure. Good carbs possess certain key traits that must be taken into consideration while incorporating them into your diet.

It is fairly easy to distinguish between good and bad carbohydrates by following a couple of pointers. For instance, anything that is organic and has been picked fresh from a garden or a farm and hasn't undergone processing would fall under the category of good carbs. Apple consumed in its original form is a good source of carbohydrates. But the juice drawn out of it after processing would make it a refined form. Therefore, they are not suitable for your diet. Even in the case of rice, brown rice is considered extremely healthy, but anything made out of it, for example, rice crackers, is processed. Therefore, they fall under the category of refined carbohydrates.

However, an exception to this rule applies when we consider the case of whole wheat pasta.

When you consume foods that are derived from the soil, it is ensured that you're eating whole foods. Things that must be included in your diet are beans, vegetables, fruit, whole grains, and so on. These foods contain copious amounts of vitamins, minerals, and a plethora of other nutrients. Fruits and vegetables have been considered to possess thousands of bioactive compounds according to scientific research. The benefits of these foods are being currently deliberated for gaining more information in scientific discourse.

The natural richness in fiber is a telling factor when it comes to the identification of good carbs. It is important to understand the details that construct the world naturally. Foods that are available in supermarkets are more often than not labeled as natural products, except in actuality their contents are highly processed. This happens because processing strips the food of all its rich natural fibers. Therefore, you must not let the sham that advertising creates misguide you in your dieting process.

There are products such as energy bars and cereals that are available at every supermarket. They are often marketed as healthy, but they are highly processed foods that can be labeled as bad carbs. The worst part about these products is that these are not only advertised incorrectly but are pumped with chemical supplements by manufacturers to make up for the nutritional value. Consumers are often unable to differentiate between these synthetic supplements and the natural ones that they require for the success of their diet plans.

According to research, fiber-rich food is considered healthy by studies that make them the focal point of their insights. The research does not include the health benefits of any kind of fibers that are included in supplements. Therefore, you cannot be sure of any health benefits accruing out of them on consumption.

However, certain categories of foods such as vegetables, whole fruit, and cooked whole grains are considered extremely profuse with natural fibers. They help to aid with cholesterol reduction, improving blood sugar levels and ensuring that you feel energetic without consuming excessive calories. In the case of other diets, the perpetual feeling of hunger persists even after consuming meals. Problems such as hemorrhoids and constipation are tackled well by the maintenance of a diet that is rich in fibers.

There are studies that suggest individuals who have higher amounts of fiber in their food are about twenty percent less likely to suffer from Type 2 diabetes. People suffering from metabolic syndrome, which is a pre-diabetic condition, can gain immense health benefits such as weight loss from including fibers in their diet. A study was conducted on those people and concluded that the incorporation of fiber in their diet helped them increase their health levels.

These results were achieved by incorporating whole foods rich in natural fibers into their diet. They were to consume foods such as vegetables and fruits that fall under the category of whole foods and contain at least thirty grams of natural fiber. They did not engage in any sort of portion control or calorie counting. Therefore, they achieved these results by simply incorporating healthy sources of carbs in their diets.

The adoption of this diet for an entire year aided these people in lowering their cholesterol levels, along with controlling their blood sugar and inflammation. The power of whole foods is evident in the health benefits these people enjoyed after the incorporation of whole foods into their diet. Weight loss is often approached in unhealthy and complex ways.

This diet, however, maintains simplicity and guarantees usefulness at the same time. Dieting can often prove to be an extremely mentally taxing exercise because complex dieting strategies often leave the person physically and mentally exhausted.

Experts suggest incorporating at least 35 to 50 grams of natural fiber in their diet on a daily basis. One must also track their fiber consumption by estimating the quantities of fiber in the food they consume. An example of this would be one cup of raw vegetables or fresh fruits would contain around two to three grams of fiber. In the case of legumes, once cooked they would consist of approximately four to seven grams of fiber.

Another way to identify good carbs is to consider the amount of water a particular food item consists of. This happens because good carbs are often rich in water content and aid hydration of the metabolic system. These foods are specifically beneficial for people aiming to lose weight and burn excess amounts of fat through the process of carb cycling.

Physically, the foods seem to be quite large in portion size, yet the calorie content is much lower as compared to other processed foods. Such foods that have large portions and low-calorie content. They also aid in the satiation of hunger, giving you a full feeling. This prevents individuals from overeating, which is a general cause of weight gain. At the same time, this fixes the problem of hunger while following a strict diet.

The composition of these foods is due to the fact that the calories that could be present in these foods are replaced by fiber and water content. This ensures that one gets to eat food that fills up their stomach, but at the same time does not promote fat accumulation.

An example of such a fruit would be watermelon that is fresh, rich in water, and calorie-free to a point where a pound of it barely consists of 300 calories. In the case of dried fruit, however, due to low water content, there is almost a 1300 calorie difference for each pound that is consumed. Dry cereal too consists of a large amount of calories, reaching 1700 calories for each pound. Therefore, foods rich in water are healthier and also rich in fiber. They possess negligible amounts of fat that also help with avoiding fat accumulation in the body.

Earlier in this book, we discussed the dangers of refined carbs. However, it must be reiterated that according to studies on carbohydrates, it is shown that refined carbs are one of the very major causes that lead to diabetes and obesity in consumers. They also create a stark imbalance in blood sugar. This is why it is important to remember that all carbs aren't beneficial.

There is an important health difference between refined and whole carbs that must not be forgotten. Therefore, this debunks the myth that all carbohydrates are sources of unhealthiness. If you want to accrue benefits out of the consumption of carbs, you must replace refined carbs with real carbs. The other options available to you are whole carbs that will help you maintain health and regulate your carb cycle according to your specific needs. This will have a long-term impact on aiding the prevention of diseases and maintaining a stable metabolism.

Fruits and Vegetables

The most important aspect of a carb cycling diet is the consumption of macronutrients. That is why it encourages you to have a plant-based diet. These diets are rich in natural carbohydrates and act as important nutrition sources for the body. Examples of consumable plant-based products are whole foods that include beans, legumes, root plants, and so on. Consumption of fruit is also central to a carb cycling diet plan, most important for higher carb days.

Plant-based diets are also among the healthiest consumable goods available in the world. This is due to the fact that they are brimming with water, dietary fibers, and antioxidants. These are very important nutrients for the body as in a diet it is very important to feel satiated. The biggest drawback of a regimented diet plan is often the client's struggle with the feeling of constant hunger. Foods that are rich in natural fiber act as great sources of nutrition. This makes them extremely important for the process of weight loss. Since they consider antioxidants, their consumption is also supposed to consist of anti-aging properties.

There are certain fruits that can be of special significance to food consumption during the process of carb cycling. They are discussed below and should be considered as important substitutes to unhealthy foods that we often consume without realizing the harmful impact in can have on our body.

Acorn Squash

All vegetables that are consumable are healthy to eat. For instance, one of the great sources of carbs is acorn squash. It has the ability to supply the body with a third of its entire day's total fiber requirement in one serving. This vegetable is immensely helpful for boosting fat-burning activity in the body at the time of exercise and also acts as a great source of vitamin C for the body.

Whole Fruit

Another vital source of good carbs is found in whole fruit. These include fruit such as blueberries and strawberries that act as brilliant antioxidants. Sweets are a very essential part of food, and fruit act as naturally grown desserts if you have a sweet tooth during your carb cycle. The source of sweetness is fructose that is naturally found in sweets. Apart from this, there are some real health benefits attached to the consumption of fruit since it are great sources of vitamins, minerals, fiber, and, most importantly, water. This water aids in hydration of the body that is extremely important in the carb dieting cycle.

Banana

Although low carb diets sometimes advise against consuming fruit, its ability to provide the body with a natural and swift boost of energy is indispensable. You might struggle with water retention and gastrointestinal issues that are addressed by consuming fruit such as bananas. Bananas have a low glycemic index, but they have high amounts of calcium and glucose. They considerably help to reduce bloating in the belly if consumed daily. Some research suggests bananas can aid in the reduction of acid reflux. Bananas also provide much-needed potassium.

Cherry

Another example of a fruit that hastens the process of weight loss is cherry. It is often referred to as a superpower fruit. The cherry's ability to act as an appropriate food during carb cycling is attributed to the richness of phytonutrient found in it.

Legumes and Tubers

Legumes

One of the most indispensable sources of fiber in a diet are legumes. Therefore, their incorporation in a carb cycling diet becomes extremely important. Legumes are rich in multiple nutrients such as proteins, fiber, and, most importantly, good carbohydrates. They create a feeling of satiation for a long time after consumption. Their central task is their ability to reduce cholesterol. If you want to lose belly fat over time, legumes are great to add to your diet.

Tuber

Tubers are a great low carb substitute for potatoes. They are infused with rich fiber and the vital nutrients necessary for a successful carb cycle. They are a type of root vegetable and they contain reserves of nutrients acquired from the underground roots of the plant.

They are incredible for digestion because they make your gut healthy. Speculated benefits range from having a role in lowering blood sugar levels and possessing anti-cancer properties.

The purpose of this section was to debunk the myths surrounding the harmful properties carbohydrates are believed of possessing.

However, a proper differentiation between refined and unrefined carbs is important to understand which source of carbohydrates you must incorporate into your carb cycling diet.

There are a plethora of organic carbohydrate sources available in the world. However, it is important to consume foods that suit your body and your carb cycling goal.

A Short message from the Author

Hey, are you enjoying the book? I would love to hear your thoughts!

Many readers do not know how hard reviews are to come by, and how much they help an author.

I would be incredibly thankful if you could take just 60 seconds to write a brief review on Amazon, even if it is just a few sentences!

Thank you for taking the time to share your thoughts!

Your review will genuinely make a difference for me and help gain exposure for my work.

Yours sincerely, John Carver

Chapter Seven:
Macronutrients and Body Systems

Carb cycling as an approach is not effective for people who are clueless about their body and the way it functions. This includes everything from knowing your body stats to knowing your allergies, the foods that you prefer, your BMI, and your glucose level. Monitoring forms a huge part of the carb cycling method and there is really no point to doing this diet in case you cannot commit to monitoring your health regularly and frequently.

There are many monitoring aids, and you must teach yourself the methods. For example, knowing that BMI needs to be considered with body fat means that you must make sure you have access to both a weight scale and a body fat scale in order for the result to be read as accurately as possible in terms of how it indicates our real health status.

You can purchase a home machine to calculate your glucose levels. Knowing how much sugar you have in your body at different parts of the diet will also give you a better idea of how the diet works and how the different levels of sugars make you feel energetic or lethargic at different points in time.

The other kind of monitoring, which is extremely important, is the nutritional value of food. While, for many foods, mainly processed ones, all nutritional information can be found on their labels, for organic food you must find them on the internet and scale it to the serving size of your choice.

Apart from being empirically important to calculating your progress within carb cycling, constant monitoring also has a radical psychological impact. It puts you in the habit of being aware of your body at all times so that you may more accurately identify what your body needs when it feels a certain way. If you haven't already been introduced to the language and aspects of body monitoring, carb cycling will make you aware of it.

You will be mindful of every bit of food you put in your body. There is no better way of looking at the body as a machine than to calculate what its working levels are and how they are acted upon by factors.

A crucial element to make sure your body monitoring is safe and happening within healthy bounds is to frequently consult a doctor or medical practitioner, who can confirm if your home calculations are correct. A doctor or medical practitioner can also analyze your diet better, and it is always informative to take a trip to the doctor during a high-level nutrition strategy that works in so many micro ways.

If you hit a roadblock while planning your meal and do not have any way of innovating new meals with your current restrictions, then a trip to a dietician is a must. A dietician understands all the different components of food better than you and may be able to recommend diet options that you didn't think were allowed during a carb restriction.

Monitoring your body and assessing your success also gives you the motivation to continue a certain diet because even more than visible proof, it is empirical proof that the human mind is trained to believe. Gradually, you also need to evolve your cycle as you become used to the current one. For this, it is important to chart out new goals that can only be done if you are aware of what your body's current needs are.

Fats, Carbs and Proteins

Part of gaining expertise in macro nutrition in theory and in practice is to understand the scientific composition of the three main macronutrients present in our diet—carbohydrates, proteins, and fats. They are responsible for supplying more than 90 percent of the weight of a diet and all of its energy. All of them have a different number of calories in a gram, and they also supply energy at different paces. Carbohydrates supply energy the fastest, and fats take the longest time to do so.

All of the digestive processes of the body happen in the large intestine. This is where they are broken down into fundamental units. Carbohydrates are converted to sugars, proteins to amino acids, and fats into fatty acids and glycerol. All these units of energy are used by the body for its growth and maintenance.

Carbohydrates

Carbohydrates are present in the body in the form of molecules. Based on the size of the molecules, carbs may be classified into simple and complex. This has been introduced in an earlier section and will be elucidated.

Simple carbs, such as sugar (glucose, sucrose) are smaller molecules. They are digested by the body and absorbed quickly, making them an instant source of energy. They make the level of sugar in the blood rise. They are present in the sweeteners used in baking goods, dairy products, fruit, and honey.

Complex carbohydrates are comprised of long chains of simple carbohydrates. When they are digested they must be broken into simple carbs and then absorbed by the body. This process is time taking and so they provide energy to the body slower than simple carbs. Unlike simple carbs, it is less likely that they are converted to fats. They raise blood sugar, but slower and more steadily. Wheat and other grains, pasta, potatoes and sweet potatoes, and root vegetables are all examples of complex carbs.

Carbohydrates may further be refined or unrefined. Refined carbs are carbs from which the fiber and minerals have been removed through processing. They are easily digested and absorbed and have little to no nutritional value. Their consumption increases the risk of weight gain and diabetes. Unrefined carbohydrates are carb rich foods in their natural state.

Proteins

When amino acids are chained together in complex formation, they form proteins. They occur in complex molecules, hence take longer to digest. They digest more slowly than carbohydrates and provide energy for a much longer period. Out of the total amino acids, the body produces some of them naturally and some must be consumed in the diet. For different proteins, there are different percentages of protein that the body can use.

Mostly, protein is used as a nutrient for growth and maintenance. However, if the body does not receive energy from elsewhere, then it is used for energy. Protein can be found in large quantities in the body since it is the primary building material for cells. Even then, if the amount of protein consumed is too much for the body, it is stored in the fat cells. 60 grams of proteins for adults and a little more for children and adults who are trying to gain muscle are recommended.

Fats

Fats, like proteins, are complex carbs; they are made up of fatty acids and glycerol. They are used for energy and to synthesize substances the body needs. There are two times more calories in a gram of fat than there are in a gram of carbohydrates or proteins. They are very slow to break down into energy and it is deposited in the body, under the skin as a reserve for when the body needs more energy.

Primarily there are three types of fats–monounsaturated fats, polyunsaturated fats, and saturated fats.

Monitoring

It is essential to the success of the carb cycling diet that you take an inventory of your body and calculate all the basic data about its levels. This must be done at least weekly if not every few days. Without the aspect of monitoring, carb cycling will not be able to create all the benefits it has the potential to create. If you are not sensitive to the changing composition of your body, you will not be able to challenge it as your diet evolves. There are two fundamental aspects to monitoring.

The first is to monitor all the basic rates of your body. These include BMI, body fat, blood glucose level, and body weight. Various tools can be used to measure these stats. The choice of whether you want to test everything at home and use certified charts to map out an idea of your body yourself or whether you want to get expert help by going to the doctor. Each approach has its pros and cons. Doing it at home yourself is the best way to increase your basic knowledge of your body and the world of health because it verses you with all the terminology and the premises that any fitness buff would be expected to have.

It is also easier to stay at home and do tests since it does not require the hassle of scheduling an appointment and does not interfere too much with your schedule. On the flip side, you might miss out on crucial signs that the body is giving you if you don't visit a doctor every few weeks because there is only a level to which a non-doctor can gain expertise on the body. Doctors also tend to have all the tools required to make testing easier, and the trip to the doctor may end up saving you the time and energy you would require to take and read the same test at home.

The second is monitoring your diet. This can be trickier than monitoring your body because your diet comprises of many complex foods that all have varying nutritional capacity. They must be calculated and synthesized to know whether you are within your calorie intake limit. There is no shortcut to knowing the number of calories in your dinner without breaking it down into its individual components, accounting for cooking methods and then calculating the calorie value of a meal yourself.

You must learn to be aware of food not just as it is prepared but also in its natural state. It helps to take your time while grocery shopping to pick out the healthiest version of what you want to consume. If your larder is stocked with healthy diet foods, then it is more freedom to experiment with meals because you know that just one ingredient will not throw your diet balance out of the window.

In principle, being aware of your body is what allows you to make variations in your diet and exercise regimens for your own betterment.

Tools

There are any tools that will aid you in the monitoring aspect and make it easier to keep track of your fitness statistics.

Body fat scales

One of the simplest methods to measure the effect of a diet is to occasionally calculate your body fat percentage. While they are not completely foolproof, you can still get an idea of what your body fat percentage is. Body fat scales comprise of a surface you simply step upon, and the machine calculates your body fat percentage for you. They have sensors inside the scale that are directly under your feet. The moment you get on the scale, an electrical current goes up the leg and pelvis. Fat is measured by looking at the amount of resistance encountered by the current from the fat present in the body. Depending on the kind of body fat scale you are using, this information will either be delivered to a smartphone or a watch. While the body fat scales can only provide rough estimates, it is still advisable to use them to measure your progress.

BMI calculator

As discussed earlier, your BMI reveals whether you are in a healthy weight range. The amount of fat around your waist is an indicator of the health risks you could face. There are many online portals available where one can calculate their BMI. The National Institute of Health has an online BMI calculator. All you need to do is to measure your height and weight in pounds and feet respectively, and the machine does the rest. This is the scale that is provided to measure the range of BMI you are in:

<18.5 = Underweight

18.5-24.9 = Normal

25-29.9 = Overweight

>30 = Obese

If a person's BMI is outside the range that is normal or healthy, the risk of many diseases goes up significantly because carrying excessive fat on your body can lead to heart problems, cardiovascular diseases and high blood pressure. Having too little weight can cause malnutrition and weak bones.

Calorie information

One of the basic limits to uphold within carb cycling is the number of calories that are consumed in a day. Hence it is very important to know the number of calories present in different foods. There are many ways to approach calorie counting. The first is to draw up a basic calorie intake limit for you based on your body weight and other factors. While preparing your meal plan, look carefully at what comprises the bulk of your diet. Draw up a calorie chart per serving of these ingredients. Divide your daily calories into many different parts based on how you plan on consuming your meals throughout the day. A low calorie group of foods can be a light breakfast and a higher calorie group can be eaten before workouts. Calorie information for most food is available online. Some producers also attach the calories per serving to products like fruit, oil, dairy and nuts. You may keep a diary of the calorie levels of the food you like to consume. This way there is a handy guide always ready to help you meal prep.

Food labels

Most processed food has a label on the packaging that contains nutritional information about the product. Information including energy or calories in kilojoule and kilocalories is usually present. Information about the amount of fat, carbohydrates, sugar, salt, and protein will also be found here. All of the information on the label corresponds to 100 grams of the product. Hence, all of your calculations must be mindful of this percentage.

There are also a few standard warning limits that let you know whether a food is too unhealthy to consume. If it has more than 17 or less than 3 grams of fat per 100 grams, it has an unhealthy amount of fat. If it has more than 22 grams but less than 5 grams of sugar per 100 grams, it has an unhealthy amount of sugars.

If it has more than 1 ½ grams or less than .3 grams of salt per 100 grams, it has an unhealthy amount of salt.

Glucometer

It is a medical device that can approximately calculate the level of glucose in the bloodstream. Home blood glucose monitoring is essential for patients with diabetes or hypoglycemia. A small drop of your blood, which can be taken by pricking your thumb with a lancet, is put on a disposable strip of glucose paper. The meter reads the strip and calculates blood glucose that is displayed in mg/dl.

Chapter Eight:
Hunger and Pleasure

At the heart of all endeavors to regulate diet as a means of body fitness, there lies a fundamental contradiction. This has been a source of anxiety for dieters for many years, and it is the reason that dieting exists and has evolved as a body of study in the last few decades. The contradiction is simply this— it has long been believed that one of the primary urges of man in nature is the urge to survive and grow.

By that logic, it can also be summarized that toward the fulfillment of the goal of survival, a living creature such as a human is willing to do whatever it takes. If there has been consensus in the world at different points of time in different eras regarding the status of some foods as good or bad, why is it that dieting as a practice needs to exist and why is it that people naturally do not gravitate toward eating whatever is healthiest for them?

Added to this, if fitness is linked to the ability of the body to survive, resist disease and protect itself against danger, why is it that the consumption of unhealthy foods is steadily on the rise?

The answer is this. Humans, considered to be at the peak of the evolutionary scale, are not merely primal animals. It is not only the basic needs of hunger and thirst that drives them to develop their dietary habits but the force of their mind and how it can persuade the body to desire foods that are explicitly unhealthy for them.

The psychology of humans is such that the mind can take over the connection of the person's behavior to their body. It can manipulate the body to participate in behaviors, which will only lead to its own destruction.

To illustrate, although it has been discovered that the creation of large-scale fast food chains is one of the primary reasons for the growing obesity in the world (which is a statistically proven fact) or that the consumption of excessively-packaged foods has increased the risk of developing cardiovascular diseases over the last few years (another proven fact), it has not led to a mass decline in the demand for these fast foods. While the body and the science around it may completely warn against certain foods, the mind is being acted upon by forces of desire for foods that are advertised to it. Since the concept of hunger is not purely physical but also includes very subjective human elements such as satisfaction and temperament, it must be studied as such in dietary research.

Where most diets fail is in accounting for the psychological pressures that the mind goes through during a certain diet. The pure restriction does not do away with the urge to consume unhealthy foods, but only shames and represses it. Hence, the concept of a cheat day in modern-day dieting has gained such massive popularity because not only does it allow for a safety valve to existing for the mental appetite of the body but also creates an incentive system that the individual can rely on to keep their investment in fitness alive.

It is in carb cycling that one can perfectly observe the kind of scientific mind-body nexus that is required for the new age dieter to truly embrace healthy life choices in a consumption culture filled with temptations and plenty of products to satiate the appetite.

Most of our eating habits are a direct result of the logic that we internalize in a market-driven world. This logic often tells us that our satisfaction is not limited to our body needs and must only be fulfilled if there are larger portions, better deals, and more variety of fried food to choose from.

It is hardly deniable that even those who embark on fitness journeys do not as much do so out of naturally wanting to be fitter, but out of the urge to train the mind not to make unhealthy choices.

It requires an iron-will and immense self-discipline, and any diet that is followed is an exercise in abstinence and deprivation. This common conception of diets can be very intimidating and makes people reject the whole idea of a healthy life because they believe that an enjoyable life should not be one based on deprivation.

Since humans are inclined to do what feels good physically, but also what feels good emotionally, it is important that the reality of the diet accommodate for both these powerful and sometimes opposing urges.

Satisfaction

There has been a discussion in the previous chapters on the aspect of refeeding days, which can become refueling days for the psyche of the dieters. Let us analyze the way this works and the impact it creates in terms of generating satisfaction for the individual who has decided to commit to a long and difficult task.

This analysis will also help us understand the purpose of refeeding days as not just simple dietary tools but an alternative way of thinking about weight loss and diets.

What is the kind of dissatisfaction that is most common in people who go on certain diets?

It is the frustration of seeing people around you consume the foods that you physically and culturally have come to love and not be able to consume them.

Our ability to eat foods also occupies a very social space in our lives. It can easily dampen the burning urge to reduce weight and causes weakness and lack of faith in the process in which one is involved. Thus, in carb cycling, there is a large pool of foods that one may choose and prepare for themselves and consume. The days you consume a high carb meal, you also don't have to suffer from the unnecessary guilt of having cheated on a diet. You already know that on those days you will end up burning more calories.

The second kind of dissatisfaction is time-bound. The gratification received from eating one meal of junk food is instant. It amplifies the temptation simply because the incentive to not eat it will not give gratifying results as quickly.

In simple words, it is easier to eat junk than to stick to a diet because while eating a packet of fries will give you immense satisfaction right now, not eating it will not show as a benefit on you instantly. Often it is a long and arduous process to visible results through dieting.

Carb cycling deals with that in two ways.

First, the entire purpose of the carb cycling approach is that it speeds up the rate at which your diet-exercise regimen can show you results. It does not allow for the body to falter, exhaust itself, or become complacent since it functions in a cyclical pattern. The individual remains enchanted with their fitness goals because they visibly see themselves gaining muscle, looking toned, and feeling better. This sense of fitness is crucial because common diets can often exhaust and starve people. It would be very difficult to stick to any life choice if it was not enjoyable and did not yield the results you wanted.

Second, the ability to gratify yourself from a meal is in no way eliminated from your life. The control, however, is passed from the hands of food chains to you yourself. A hearty breakfast does not always have to be fried foods but can also be a rich bowl of oatmeal and fresh fruit.

Fish, chicken, and other proteins are not excluded from the diet, and there is a constant incentive to innovate. It also helps to put the order of priorities in perspective. Feeling hungry for a delicious meal does not have to mean that you end up eating junk food. It simply means you need to look twice at your options and pick the healthier ones. Once this kind of logic is accepted, you are all set for a lifetime of making healthier choices and not compromising on the pleasure you derive from food.

To get the most out of your diet, you must learn how to get the most out of your refueling experience. On high carb days, you have a lot of freedom to design your meals. Here you can experiment with different ingredients and cooking styles available to you and add as much variety to your meals as possible. This must also be psychologically reinforced as a well-made, well-deserved meal because it is preceded and followed by a low carb day.

Experimentation

One of the most staggering obstacles to weight loss is that all new diets and exercise fads will slow down or stop the kind of results that you can gain from them.

This phenomenon in the fitness world is known as 'weight plateau,' or in simple terms, hitting an equilibrium where your body systems have been given enough time to get used to the impact of your current diet and exercise routine.

At this point, the body regulates its metabolism to make sure that calories are not being burned at an unreasonable rate. For people dedicated to long-term weight loss, this is the most difficult period to get over since it requires an extra effort that is made out to be difficult and inaccessible to the common people. When stories float around of athletes spending twelve hours training every day, the average person immediately overvalues the kind of effort required to cross to the other side of the weight plateau.

This can be a very alienating experience for many. This is the perfect example of the mixture of physical and mental factors combining to create an impossible situation.

Carb cycling, on the other hand, poses a question to this belief. It reveals that it is not the time and energy given to a diet, but the amount of attention given to it, which determines its success. There are two aspects to this. On a primary level, carb cycling decodes the methods of athletes themselves and reveals it to be about scientific calculation as opposed to pure hard work. On a secondary level, it makes all these methods accessible to people by creating proximities with things that they are familiar with it.

Moreover, it is renewable as a dieting technique. Every time a weight plateau is reached, your metabolism can be increased again if carb cycling is duly used. It does not exhaust itself in one go but can be customized according to your needs and experiences.

It is a self-reforming dieting technique, and, in that sense, irreplaceable. It cannot be outgrown because it evolves to suit your current needs. This renewability gives it value in the age of diets that are only effective for one use.

Carb cycling can be practiced a different way every time it is renewed. Your initial goal may have been to lose weight, so you followed two low carb days a week with a cardio-intensive exercise routine. After you have lost the desired amount of weight, you can modify your diet according to your next goal. If your next goal is to gain muscle and become toned, you can incorporate more protein and weight training exercises.

There is endless freedom to experiment with a carb cycling diet.

Results and success

Where does the success of a diet lie? Weight scales don't act the same for everyone, and visible results cannot be trusted, starvation is simply bad practice–then where does one look for a metric to evaluate the quality of a diet?

The success of a diet lies in how efficiently it can persuade the individual to take care of their own body and make mindful decisions for it. A diet that offers good complete nutrition and in turn good health is always better than a diet that promises only weight loss.

In simple words, a diet that is able to make you adopt a certain lifestyle over your current one is the diet that is most effective.

Let us look at the lifestyle creation aspect of it a little deeply.

A lifestyle is not defined by one or two elements that you incorporate into your life; it is rather an attitude that determines the choices you will make concerning you and your surroundings. When you accept the lifestyle that consumer media wants to impose on you, you'll find yourself surrounded by commodities that you don't always need but are convinced you want. The same applies to your eating habits. If the notion of having a calorie intake limit is not present in the fast food market, which serves huge portions, you will also not incorporate counting calories into your lifestyle.

A lifestyle also defines your routine and the activities that utilize the most amount of time and energy in your day.

Carb cycling makes you believe in the lifestyle of fitness in two crucial ways:

Watching what you eat

On a carb cycling diet, you are required to be constantly vigilant.

Not only vigilant only about how much you consume but to also be vigilant about the nutritional composition of the various foods you are consuming. This habit of watching what you eat requires a great knowledge of food, what it contains, how it reacts with the body, and how much it contributes to or takes away from your fitness goals. Once this knowledge has been created in your mind, it will be nearly impossible for them to not apply it to everything you eat, even outside of the diet. Once you are aware that eating one hamburger may completely destroy the effect of the intense workout you did the previous day, you will definitely think twice before you eat it.

This vigilant attitude is especially beneficial for adults who are growing older since fresh eating delays the effect of aging on the body.

Believing in the power of exercise

Carb cycling reinforces the idea that for every loaded meal there must be equally intense exercise. The enjoyment food is only complete if it does not tamper with your fitness goals. Exercising may even become more fun for you because you are required to do it on the days when you have more energy to expend.

With these two elements combined, you'll have achieved the best possible lifestyle to stay fit your entire life. The success of carb cycling lies in making healthy choice natural for you. It is to incline you to be aware of what you are eating every time you eat. This, by far, is the most you can do in terms of truly taking your fitness in your own hands. It is about making the decision to not rely on internet fads but to listen to your own body.

Chapter Nine:
Implementations On Purpose

Carb cycling is used for various purposes in health and fitness. As discussed extensively in the earlier sections, this approach can affect every system of the body positively. It ranges from physical muscle development to chemical, hormonal balance, and psychological condition. It is beneficial for digestive health, blood insulin levels, dental health, and gut health. Its mass appeal is based primarily on its emphasis on body knowledge, personal physiology, and data analysis. It is an extremely high level and precise way of dieting, and gives greater control to you to customize it according to your unique needs and diet. It dispels the notion that fitness methods are universal and applicable to everyone. By taking control of the smallest aspects of this dietary approach, you take far greater control of your health and are likelier to remain invested in the cause of becoming healthier.

However, what sets this diet apart from others and makes it more effective is also what makes it incredibly difficult for some people to follow. Carb cycling requires constant monitoring of many variables and a good knowledge of your body. This is both on the level of data and intuition. It is recommended that before planning a carb cycle, people should not only be aware of preliminary bodily statistics such as weight, height, and BMI but also have a more intricate knowledge of the state of their hormones, their cholesterol levels, their blood insulin levels and their blood pressure.

All of these have to be accommodated for during the carb cycle. For example, if body cholesterol is higher, there needs to be more consumption of lean fish during the high carb days. This achieves the twin effect of balancing cholesterol while achieving your primary weight loss goal. These variables need to be frequently rechecked and accounted for in your diet and exercise schedule, which can be a tedious process for many. However, with the right amount of care and respect for your body, it can also make you get rid of the attitude of casual dieting that is not only unreliable and ineffective but also harmful for the body.

You must ensure that you are in touch with the needs of your body as they can be felt. Be vigilant for any negative changes being brought on by changes in dieting habits. On a fundamental level, this includes being careful of allergies while trying out new foods such as whole grains or nuts. It also means that care must be taken to stay adequately hydrated and full. Self-discipline regarding junk food needs to be as rigorously applied as does not overwork yourself on high carb days. It must be remembered that the body in its natural state is the healthiest, and any extreme behavior upon it can disrupt its natural functioning. You need to listen with care to the cues that the body gives you.

Body Goals

The constant monitoring that this diet demands can be quite tedious for those who are more accustomed to casual dieting. Let us look at the reality of how carb cycling looks for the individual undertaking it. On a regular day, this involves not only planning your meal beforehand but also adjusting it according to the kind of day you have ahead. Casual snacking and cheat days are to be strictly replaced with high carb days, which are equivalently monitored to ensure maximum benefit. These can involve making changes in your meal plans every few days. Combine this with the fact that this diet works principally on a fluctuating meal cycle that needs to be rigorously maintained. In simple words, it is not a straightforward diet. While this may appear discouraging to many, it is not very difficult to implement if you understand the underlying logic behind why certain meals are to be eaten at a certain time.

On an application level, this dietary approach cannot be followed blindly, and this is crucial to its success. You cannot copy a meal plan without also finding an adequate exercise routine that works simultaneously with it. This diet will also not show instant results and requires a certain amount of commitment to fitness. Some accounts found in different sources that declare this diet is not effective are actually the result of poor understanding and poor application of this diet. After going through them, a few fundamental mistakes that casual dieters often do while following this diet can be easily identified are as mentioned below.

Imitation diets

For any individual who is excited to be in a new dietary approach, a fatal flaw is to approach carb cycling the way that they would approach a traditional diet such as the grapefruit diet, which has a standard calorie intake irrespective of who practices it. In this scenario, imitating a diet can lead to detrimental results, which is that if an average person follows the meal plan of a sportsperson who is practicing carb cycling, they will end up putting on weight instead of shedding it since their calorie intake will be equal to the athlete's but their exercise routine will not.

Misidentifying good carbs and bad carbs

Unless you exhaustively go through trustworthy lists of what food products contain, you might end up incorporating processed sugars and bad carbs in your diet. While all fruits are healthy foods, bananas should not be consumed on low carb days because they are high in carbs. Even if a flawed meal plan is followed rigorously, it will not yield results if it is not allowed to work upon the body as it should. While organic oatmeal is a good breakfast for a high carb day, sugary cereal will have the opposite effect because while it is rich in carbs, it is rich in the wrong kind of carbs. It is best to eat home-prepped meals made with the freshest produce. If a fruit bowl is a good snack option, the kind of fruit it is made of also needs to change according to what carb day it is in the cycle. The same applies to everything from vegetables to meat.

Incompatible Exercise regimen

The point of consuming more carbs on certain days is to give enhanced energy for better physical performance. The high carb days must not always be treated as cheat days or refeed days because they serve a very specific kind of purpose in the carb cycle. High carb consumption needs to be accompanied by high-intensity training. If there is only moderate exercise during high carb days and high-intensity workout during the low carb ones, the cycle of fatigue and the weight plateau will continue to persist.

Impatience

The primary goal of carb cycling is not to instantly lose weight, but to eliminate all the possible reasons people do not lose weight despite eating healthy. It may almost be considered a supplementary tool, which makes weight loss techniques effective. It does not let the body turn on itself in a fitness journey. Thus, if you are not willing to move away from the narrow idea of fitness as thinness you will be able to devote the kind of trust required by this dietary method. You will enjoy not just quantitative results but qualitative ones. Losing weight without feeling toned, healthy, and fit is an outmoded idea.

You must accept that the long-term benefits carb cycling can provide cannot be reaped in a short period. A universal complaint with fad diets is that there is a considerable amount of weight gain immediately after the diet ends. Through carb cycling, you are training your body to develop the urge to exercise whenever it consumes higher carbs and to demand fewer carbs when it is at rest. This can control unhealthy eating habits for a lifetime.

Out of impatience, people do not take the time to design their meal plans in a way so they aren't denied of any of the food they like and end up putting themselves on impossible diets because it is quite difficult to stay true to a diet that you loathe. Meanwhile, those who seriously customize their meal plans include everything from avocado to beans and a selection of flavors from vegetables and fruit. Not only is a varying diet easier to follow, but also it is also more beneficial.

Diet Combination

As it must have become sufficiently clear, carb cycling is a multipurpose diet. It is not a universally standardized plan, and that is exactly what makes it so versatile in its range of applications. There is always a space within carb cycling to accommodate any other diet plans you might want to follow. Carb cycling does not require you to eliminate any particular macro nutritional food group from your diet. There is great space for a play between the elements of your preferred diet and carb cycling. Here are a few examples to illustrate.

If there is a desire in you to opt for vegetarian foods, then carb cycling encourages you to look into the different sources of your required macro nutrition doses. As opposed to protein-heavy diets that encourage meat-eating, in carb cycling you can obtain the required amount of nutrients from leafy vegetables, potatoes, legumes, and so on. Thus, a vegetarian or a vegan diet, if it is to be converted into a fitness diet and not a lifestyle choice, can be molded to function within the requirements of the carb cycle to fulfill nutritional needs.

Intermittent fasting is yet another dietary phenomenon that is gaining popularity in the fitness world. Like the term itself suggests, it entails fasting intermittently over longer periods of time. There are various popular variants of this diet, depending on the time period for which fasting is done.

The alternate-day fasting is probably the most rigorous way of intermittent fasting because it has a daylong fasting period followed by a daylong non-fasting period. Whole-day fasting requires one or two days of fasting every week. Time-restricted fasting only allows eating food for a few hours at certain points of time in the day. This is also known as the 16/8 method because it has a 16-hour fasting period and an eight-hour non-fasting period.

Intermittent fasting, again, is not a conventional diet since it does not specify what is to be eaten. Instead, it is more like an eating pattern. Since it doesn't say what to eat but only when to eat, it can be beautifully complemented by a carb cycling-based diet and exercise regimen. This is particularly true of the 16/8 method because the eight hours of eating in a day can include meals according to their respective days in the carb cycle.

The carb cycle of an intermittent faster can be specially tailored to fit the needs of their body. Insulin levels drop quite drastically when intermittent fasting, and healthy carbs can be included in the diet to balance out the process and lower insulin gradually so that the body may have more time to adjust to burning fat. In the absence of this, it is likely that you immediately regain your entire lost weight right after you stop fasting because insulin deficiency you crave unhealthy carbs.

The benefits of intermittent fasting can be accrued without experiencing the short timespan they usually manifest. The belly fat, which is one of the indicators of bad health of vital organs, is particularly targeted through intermittent fasting. If it is combined with carb cycling, then you can also incorporate muscle building and strength to this fitness plan and experience an overall rise in agility and tone.

Meal Prep

It has been emphasized that meal prep forms a fundamental part of the success of carb cycling. While it can be a very tedious task to some, there are two clear benefits.

First, lifestyle simplification is a perfectly achievable goal when you prep meals for carb cycling. Most modern lifestyles are overly complicated because of the material commodities that we surround ourselves with and spend time buying. While carb cycling, you can focus more money on buying fresh produce, which is also available for non-extravagant prices.

As opposed to this, the consumer pressure to consistently keep your shelves stocked up with items that your body does not ask for is a surefire way to normalize unhealthy eating and buying habits. Many processed foods and bad carbs also function in a way that those who consume them never feel satisfied with their meal. Through meal prepping, one can regain control of the body's unhealthy impulses.

The accumulation of materials like plastic and other packaging can be drastically reduced once diets are preplanned and not ordered or bought at a convenience store. It generates an interest in the tenet of treating one's body as a temple and only consuming the most nourishing substances for it. Once you completely believe in the logic of carb cycling, you are bound to look at food not as a guilty pleasure but as an aid in your fitness journey.

Second, it will help you build your metabolic profile. A metabolic profile reveals your ability to gain nourishment from and digest different food groups at different speeds. Since carb cycling focuses on monitoring, you can build a metabolic profile of your body's responses to different substances and not just prep meals for a few days or weeks, but make a monthly or yearly calendar. This metabolic profile reveals a lot of secret information about the body of a person and how it acts under particular circumstances. Once this is established, even a basic meal can be broken down into its different components and analyzed for their nutritional value before they are consumed.

Beyond these two general benefits, there is also the freedom to allow for different factors to be accommodated within your meal plan such as your budget, dietary preferences, the season, your fitness goals, and, most importantly, your desired foods. The body is not taught to repress the desire to eat delicious food but always to put its health as a top priority and look for healthier alternatives to their favorite foods.

Chapter Ten:
Application of Method

As discussed in earlier chapters, humans possess varying bodies with varying needs and purposes. The strategy of carb cycling works on a common formula of regulating carbs, but the method of regulation is often different for each body type. Carb cycling is practiced by common people for maintaining fitness, as well as by specialized professionals such as bodybuilders and models. There are different ways to approach carb cycling, depending on your needs and desires.

A question people often raise about carb cycling has to do with how much influence it has on muscle gain. There is a common misconception that carbs only generate fat accumulation in the body. In fact, carb cycling aids people in gaining the muscle mass they desire. In order to gain muscle through this strategy, it is important to maintain a calorie surplus.

Extensive training is a daily requirement for certain people, yet it is essential to provide your body with rest. This is important for it to recover from the intensity of the workout, and also for carb cycling to generate positive results. Another kind of training that experts suggest is resistance training. This is influenced by the fact that when the body loses weight, it cannot gain muscle. Either of those two processes cannot occur in tandem because while one needs a calorie surplus, the other needs a calorie deficit. Due to this, your carb cycling routine must be adjusted according to your lifestyle and fitness goals.

A strategic refeeding of carbs is required for gaining muscle. The tricky part of this is that a calorie surplus leads to weight gain, and fat gain along with muscle gain is inevitable. This is where the management of calories in such a way that they are enough for muscle gain but don't pose a risk of weight gain is important. Muscle gain can't be altered by a simple change in macronutrient ratio.

Method

Carb cycling is a strategy that is based on altering the number of carbs you consume every day in alternative proportions. For instance, some high carb days are mixed with low carb days in a given carb cycling week.

This alternating strategy can be adjusted according to personal fitness goals for achieving specific results.

Due to the multifaceted nature of physical types and different personal goals, there are a plethora of methods to take up carb cycling. A generalized method would be to mix low carb days, high carb days, and medium carb days according to your routine. The diet achieves its results by manipulating the number of carbs consumed each week.

Carb cycling aims to absorb all nutrients through carbohydrates. Therefore, make optimal use of every meal. This way, the body is satisfied and strong but is also not overloaded by carbs to a point where it would cause weight gain.

Application on Training Routine

The carb cycling approach can be utilized for achieving different results. Yet it is essential to grasp a general understanding of how it functions before we move on to its specific application. Let's clarify what we mean by high carb days, low carb days, and medium carb days.

Days that are referred to as high carb days can be helpful in multiple ways. There are diets, which eliminate all kinds of carbs from your routine and constantly reinforce the belief that carbs are fattening or bad for your health. The myth around reducing carb consumption for weight loss does not account for the benefits of high carb days provide. The body often loses glycogen and high carb days help in its replenishment. Some people suffer from a lack of appetite. High carbs are beneficial to fix this problem since they restore leptin in the body, which is the hunger hormone. The body is a high functioning machine, and its performance is considerably enhanced through the consumption of good carbs in large amounts.

On low carb days, the body loses a large amount of protein and high carb days help to prove this extra protein for the muscles that break down. This breakdown can occur due to intermittent fasting too. There is a common misconception around carb cycling being solely for fat reduction. It aids muscle building simultaneously, which is why it is a coveted method for bodybuilders. Therefore, it is a holistic formula for achieving fitness. The best part about a carb cycling diet is that it allows you to live your life as you want and does not restraint you like other diets. It is merely built around following a systematic carb consumption routine along with ensuring that the food consumed does not fall in the category of refined carbohydrates.

To paint a picture of a usual high carb day, you must imagine meals, which are made up of more than fifty percent of macronutrients derived by carbohydrates. As discussed earlier, whole food, fruit, and starch consumption will be amped up considerably. This will be based on your personal requirements and routine. On high carb days specifically, consumption of around 220 - 440 carbs is considered legitimate. Anyone engaged in intensive exercise and training should participate at the higher end of this spectrum. Others should stick to the 220 grams a day. Workouts that are of a high-intensity nature require 440 gm carbs. Cardio, on the other hand, can make do with 220 gm.

One of the many questions that people are planning to undertake carb cycling is the amount of fat loss one can achieve through it. There's a positive answer to this, and it is a fact that carb cycling aids weight loss. It differs from other diets in its methodology, which is what makes it a unique strategy of dieting. The prerequisite for fat loss is achieving a calorie deficit. In other words, your ability to burn fat must trump your consumption. In a scenario where this doesn't happen, fat accumulation begins. Carb cycling makes weight loss possible by making sure that you feel satisfied on days labeled as high carb days.

This is balanced out by medium and low carb days. Since carbohydrates are an excellent source of energy, such a balancing out ensures that you have plenty of it while going on with your daily life. Training is not hindered by this diet since it doesn't let the feeling of weakness or malnourishment percolate into your system. Athletes, bodybuilders, models, and other people who want their performance levels to improve will experience great results since their bodies will be pushed to burn faster while retaining their health. This is why carb cycling is often undertaken by people engaged in these professions.

In slight opposition to a high carb day, a medium carb day allows for about twenty to fifty percent macronutrient consumption through carbohydrates. A simple way to understand this quantity would be to measure carb consumption in relation to your body weight in grams. For instance, if you are a 110 pounds, your carb consumption should be around 70 - 140 on a medium carb day.

The cumulative amount of carb consumption will be contingent on the caloric requirement or the day in question. These numbers are simply an example, and they differ from person to person. The source of carbs on these days should be green vegetables and regulated portions of fruit.

The tricky area of carb cycling is making the most of low carb days. This is the day the body is supposed to generate a calorie deficit to aid weight loss. Some people who suffer from insulin spikes consider this a beneficial strategy to reduce it. Unlike high and medium carb days, low carb days would require only about ten percent of your energy sources to be derived from carbohydrates. There is also a scenario when consuming no carbs at all would be viable. This is heavily dependent on your personal body requirements and abilities. About fifty grams of carbohydrates are the highest amount of carbs you can consume if any.

Good carbohydrates can be consumed in the form of green vegetables, as preferred by people who indulge in this diet plan. It is less advisable to opt for no-carb days. If you do decide to opt for them, you must consume meals containing fat and meat. Through this, you will get your required fill of fat as well as protein. There isn't a general formula to carb cycling you must follow. It is important to keep your body and health in mind while making any decisions.

Therefore, this is the baseline you must follow for training your body in a carb cycling diet. This can be adjusted according to your body needs and plans. Each high carb and low carb day possesses its own purpose in the totality of the carb cycling process. All days work in tandem with each other, which is to say, consuming more carbs on one day and fewer carbs on another will not negate the benefits generated out of either of the days.

Carb cycling is based on the idea of creating a balance in the body. This cumulative effect of low, high, and medium carb days is what generates a healthy body.

Since this diet is carbohydrate centric, it is important to acknowledge the role of other macronutrients like protein. A ten-gram intake of protein for each pound of your weight is considered as the appropriate amount of protein you must consume. For instance, if you weigh 110 pounds, you must consume 110 grams of protein to maintain the balance. This consumption pattern for protein is generally static for almost everybody. When it comes to fat, about fifteen to 35 percent of your total calories must be derived from its consumption in your diet.

Athletic Fueling

Carbohydrates are one energy source that athletes rely heavily on for meeting their energy requirements on a daily basis. Due to this, ketogenic diets seem extremely difficult to follow in their pursuit of health and fitness. For those indulging in exercise, carbohydrates are considered the most important nutrient to derive energy. There needs to be consistency between their diet and training regime for achieving body goals. Carb cycling can have multiple benefits, which include altering body composition, improving performance and recovery, keeping metabolic health in check, and so on.

As discussed earlier, low carb days form an important part of the carb cycling process. It is scientifically conjectured that training on low carb days aids in weight loss, boosts the burning of body fat considerably, and also results in speeding up aerobic adaptation required for training. Athletes encounter a conundrum in this scenario because they need a high amount of carbohydrates to fuel their intensive training and want to gain benefits of carb regulation and restriction at the same time. To keep the system working well, the diet must be adjusted according to athletic requirements. For instance, the upper limit of carbohydrate consumption on a high carb day will apply to a person going through training and exercise.

Athletes need to make sure that their body has enough carbs for performance in training; otherwise, it can be detrimental to their health. Since the nature of the exercise is tough, the body needs to stock up on carbohydrates on these days. It is advised to consume carbs before a workout because they are the most instant source of energy for fueling intensive physical activity.

It does not enable the body to indulge in a short duration workout, which is high in intensity. An interesting fact to note about carbohydrates is that even in the absence of ingestion when it is still in the human mouth, it generates benefits like increase in performance capabilities due to the activation of certain regions of the brain that aid in motor control.

Heavy exercising and training require a period of rest for the body to recover from the rigorous routine it has to go through. Carbohydrates are a great source to hasten the process of recovery. Post-exercise consumption of carbohydrates has the ability to synthesize protein and glycogen resynthesize. Performance and recovery, the two essential elements of physical training become improved due to the process of carb cycling. Days that require a high quality of physical response become an easier reality when athletes follow this strategy of dieting.

Competitions

Carb cycling is often used to prepare bodies for partaking in competitions such as bodybuilding. Athletes engaging in this diet for preparing their bodies for participation need to make sure that they reduce their calorie intake in phases. They must also follow a strictly controlled meal preparation plan. Their calorie intake should be cycled, as done through carb cycling in the form of high, medium, and low carb days. Athletes also often make mistakes while dieting, such as reducing calorie intake suddenly. This leads to an imbalance in the metabolism that hampers long-term results. Therefore, they need to be aware of the mistakes they make in a dieting plan.

The first advice would be to phase their calorie intake down. There are people who often employ more than one diet to achieve bulking. They ignore the fact that the increase in calories should be slow and gradual for bulking, and the decrease should be the same while cutting. Diets that are altered overnight often result in excessive weight gain while trying to bulk, which defeats the purpose of the diet. A sudden decrease in calories leads to muscle loss and becomes counterproductive for your goals as it does not achieve cutting.

Calorie intake must be adjusted by 150 grams each week. This step is important for the body to adjust to the changing nutrition conditions. It helps to maintain the muscle mass they so desperately require. It would be disastrous for a bodybuilder, for instance, to lose all the weight they wanted only to realize that they've lost muscle mass as well. This is why the importance of phasing must be reiterated.

During the course of dieting, you must avoid making approximations. Every calorie reduction should be measured in their exact amounts and reduced or increased. For example, 150 gram reduction shouldn't be one based on approximation.

The most important part of preparation is the cycle of calorie intake. Many opinions exist on the matter of how to regulate calorie intake. But there's an overwhelming consensus on cycling as the best option for achieving the desired results.

The metabolism instantly speeds up the moment there is a significant increase in calorie intake on a given day. This makes space for the body to allow an easy way to achieve a calorie deficit on the following days of the cycle. Benefits of high carb days include the increase of strength levels, due to the refueling of glycogen levels in the muscle that improve energy.

It is advised to follow a six-day consistent diet plan in a carb cycling week, with one day as the high carb day. The day that requires the highest physical activity should be considered as the high carb day.

Chapter Eleven:
Monitoring and Coaching

The prerequisite for following any diet is ensuring that it is medically viable. Much like any other diet, carb cycling entails strategic alterations in your nutritional lifestyle, which have long-term impacts on your physical and mental health. It is advised to consult your nutritionist before undertaking a regimented diet to ensure that it is safe to do so. They must be presented with your medical history consisting of both past and current medical records.

Once your diet is sanctioned by the doctor or the health expert, constant monitoring is important to maintain safety and effectiveness.

The monitoring process must be undertaken by you personally on a regular basis. At the same time, you must seek professional help for being up to date with your progress. This professional help exists in the form of methodologies, such as food coaching and medical monitoring. Once you've decided to undergo the process of carb cycling, the first step is to consult a food coach who can draw up a proper routine and distinct strategy for your unique needs. It also helps to build knowledge about your body and making you adept enough to serve yourself properly during the course of the diet.

Since calorie intake influences hormonal changes, alters glycogen levels, metabolism speed and general bodily functions, it is important to monitor your body's response constantly. It is essential to do so to not only ensure medical safety but also to track your body's gradual progress. Tracking changes in your body will help you boost your morale since diets can often prove to be difficult to maintain. You will see physical changes only after a considerable amount of time; therefore, only monitoring can ensure you're up to date with your body's health status.

Carb cycling diets need to be altered as the days progress to keep up with the changes in the body. Monitoring is essential to update your carbohydrate intake plan and to ensure it doesn't lose its effectiveness as time passes.

Food Coaching

An individual's potential to identify healthy food choices and prioritize their wellbeing through every stage of their lives is one that must be harnessed. This is precisely what food coaching aims to achieve. It comes under the category of health coaching and aids individuals to progress in their fitness journeys. Aimed at ensuring appropriate food consumption and preventing diet-related diseases, it is enshrined in the principles of interdisciplinary, science-based methodology.

Food coaching is a method to gain advanced knowledge about the diets we undertake. It isn't a mere source of generalized dietary recommendations and basic health coaching. It trains people to interact with the details of their daily consumption patterns. By being more in touch with how food affects you, you will be adept letting your optimal self-shine through.

The methodology in the discussion is a food-focused practice that is part of a highly specialized category of food-based coaching. It ensures fulfillment of long-term goals that aid in maintaining flourishing health and wellbeing. The variety of information it helps to impart include a detailed understanding of figuring out food preferences, food preparation, food selection, and storage.

Food coaching works on the principle, which prioritizes the promotion of your wellbeing. People often neglect to adhere to the fitness recommendations that are made by their doctors and nutritionists. In this scenario, it is important for you to engage in the enhancement of your attention to health practices. Dietary patterns could seem like something you can figure out for yourself, but this is a myth. This myth can be transformed into reality only through the help of food coaching, which lays down rules, regulations, and guidelines for healthy interaction with food. Especially in the case of carb cycling, it is important to incorporate such strategies to prevent a plethora of diseases and health risks.

One of the central environmental factors that people are forced to on a daily basis is their dietary pattern. The diet is an environmental factor. It is something that people can be taught to control from an early age to ensure that they do not fall prey to any diet-related diseases. Unhealthy living conditions that may trigger side effects like aging.

This fact has been legitimized by referring to RCT (randomized, and controlled intervention) trials which depicted that adherence to dietary patterns could lead to primary prevention of cardiovascular diseases.

Healthcare practitioners continue to struggle with ensuring adherence to healthy patterns of diet and lifestyles in general, despite the fact that advanced scientific guidelines for health care exist in the field.

The primary cause of illness when a person encounters a chronic disease is often lack of following healthcare guidelines, as noticed by professionals.

Whole food consumption has come to take a significant place in the conversation of a healthy lifestyle. This is since it is natural and sustainable and has become the focal point of preventive health care, and is gaining ground to become the central method of treatment in a plethora of cases. Individuals are often unaware of how they are to choose and find the right kind of food to eat. This problem persists to a point where people are often also unaware of what kind of food may have scientific benefits and how they are to be incorporated in their diet.

We live in an era of information, and you can find sources to deal with your unawareness. Due to the lack of accountability and generalized nature of this information, you might feel lost about how to apply this in your daily lives. This misinformation is often expressed in the form of a lack of knowledge of the appropriate quality and quantity of the food you need to consume. Quantities can greatly influence the entire effect of the diet.

For instance, carb cycling is based on the principle of high, low, and medium carb days, which are largely determined by specific quantities decided by taking body type, BMI, etc. into consideration. This problem is also specific to whole food consumption.

To overcome this complexity, people often turn to misinformation from unreliable online sources to find quick and easy fixes. These methods, if not all, at least the majority of them are absent of any scientific precision, basis, and education in the theory of food selection. The importance of food quality cannot be overstated as it allows us to repair, heal, and find molecular and genetic balance. However, it is unfortunate that this information often doesn't get transmitted to the customer.

Food coaching can help you achieve all your fitness goals by making you aware of the many details that eating consist of. It trains you to reorient your everyday live according to scientific evidence by providing with the knowledge of what can be beneficial for you. It aims to help you to rethink the idea of food itself and reorganize your life according to the newfound knowledge base. This is especially true for whole foods.

The priorities of food coaching are; facilitation of knowledge, enhancement of behavioral change in lieu of consumption choices, and elimination of innate frustrations that people possess due to dieting.

The whole job of food coaches is to make support available to the client in order to enhance their chances of achieving appropriate goals. The sessions are generally spaced into one class a week, but could also be spaced further into being once every two weeks. This is contingent on the client and their preferences and needs.

One of the primary responsibilities of a food coach is to respect and prioritize the values that are important to the client when it comes to food concerns. This is attributed to the fact that people possess different lifestyles influenced by religious and cultural practices. People who seek more balanced options, often aim their energies at redefining what essentially a quality of life means for them. Since values are inherent and exercise immense control over our primary life principles, they may serve as a motive for individuals to make healthy choices, accomplish tasks, and challenge tricky situations. Therefore, our values have a strong effect on our motivations.

While the process of food coaching is going on, it is absolutely essential to understand the specific facts behind food behavior and control them enough so you can relate it to motivation. Motivation can only be internalized when personal goals are linked to personal values that form our will and spirit for achievement.

Medical Monitoring

In a diet strategy like carb cycling, it is important to monitor and measure progress. Currently, there aren't any strategies that measure dietary intake accurately. Methodologies that currently exist to measure food consumption consist of high inaccuracy rates. Despite this, measuring nutritional intake accurate is a prerequisite to track nutritional status, monitor the needs of a population, and gauge the effectiveness of interventions by the state through public nutritional health policies. To achieve this end, it is essential to develop methods that facilitate proper and accurate assessment of a population's nutritional intake without having too much of an effect on their daily routines.

This is more of a holistic understanding of measuring overall nutritional intake. However, currently, we're discussing more individualized instances of measurement. In a diet such as a carb cycling, monitoring is important to measure the application of the diet plan. Monitoring also aids in realizing the amount of progress you have made by virtue of the diet. In the previous section, we discussed the importance of staying motivated through our diet. Tracking progress helps us in ensuring that we feel motivated since we understand the kind of changes our body is going through.

In the process of medical monitoring, one can make charts, schedule monthly check-ups, or even keep constant track by the help of information technology-based solutions.

One of the most millennial formulations of medical monitoring at home is the development of apps.

Diet Monitoring Apps

In a carb cycling diet, constant monitoring is important. Since it works on a formula of combining different carb days. It also needs to be regimented in order to work appropriately. To make healthier food decisions and to eat the right kind of food, it is important for you to keep track of what you consume each day. Tracking your diet without any external help is not easy. But once you've made this decision to commit to your diet, you need to get hold of a tracking tool. Such tracking tools exist in the most accessible forms through apps that you can download on your device. Tools are incredible at making it possible for you to chart what you consume, add, subtract, and eliminate calories, or save up information about your nutrition intake can help you work toward achieving your goals.

A list of few nutrition trackers will be discussed below, which will help you choose an appropriate diet-monitoring app for your carb cycling journey.

My Fitness Pal

To access one of the largest food databases available in a diet tracking app, which is available as a website, as well as being available on your Android or Apple device, you must check out MyFitnessPal. It has a plethora of choices for your exclusive needs. Whether you're cooking at home or going out for lunch, it helps you sort your diet according to your schedule.

It can help you list all the carbs you have consumed in a day and log the food you've consumed.

It consists of a list of restaurant menus so you can access any kind of food as per your indoor and outdoor needs. Once you sign in, you can get a holistic picture of your dietary practices along with your overall calorie consumption. You can track your cholesterol consumption, sodium consumption, vitamin consumption and information about other nutrition you consume, which can help you gauge your dieting lifestyle more than a mere calorie restriction.

The additional benefit it possesses is the community of people who you can interact with on your dieting journey. Here you can interact and gain from the knowledge that people share on dieting tricks, meal plans, recipes, and stories of success or disappointment with different nutritional practices.

The best part about this application is that it's completely free. Apart from being accessible, it also syncs external activity trackers and apps you might already be referring to.

It helps to monitor as it doesn't push a particular dieting agenda on its users. It's aimed at being a database for tracking nutrition and comes with the added benefit of a wholesome community that helps you keep your motivation intact.

LoseIt

It is important to have a tracker that tracks food and physical activity, and LoseIt combines both of those features. It has enjoyed popularity among individuals who are trying to track their weight loss journeys, calorie goals, and consumption, and generally pay attention to the nature of the foods they eat.

As well as having a website application, it too has an Android and Apple version with the added benefit of a barcode that can scan the packaged food you consume and display the appropriate servings or the ingredients you need for preparing dishes.

The LoseIt community is a helpful one when it comes to tracking your fitness goals and making sure you're following your diet without fail.

SparkPeople

SparkPeople is an application that allows multiple sites to form a network. Its central aims are rooted toward helping people live healthier lives. Each site that forms a part of the

SparkPeople network is aimed at different areas of your health and wellness concerns.

It is a very efficient nutritional intake tracker, and it also helps individuals in tracking the physical activity they've engaged in over a day.

In terms of nutrition, it helps you track your daily food consumption in the form of meals, make a list of the food you've cooked yourself, and also access restaurant items.

All this information is accumulated and then broken down to provide you with a complete picture of your nutritional practices.

Specifically, for the purpose of carb cycling, it will aid you to track the carbs you consume along with vitamins and minerals.

It also ensures you fulfill the daily requirement of carbs, minerals, or vitamins by helping you make a list of the foods you eat. It combines the effect physical activity has on your diet. It can help you keep track of low, medium, and high carb days and gage the difference between each of them. It also makes a list of how much sugar you're consuming each day and whether you've fulfilled the daily allowance of minerals and vitamins. Its accessibility through Android and Apple smartphones ensures that you have your fitness monitor on the go.

It comes with the notification feature, which can help you set personal reminders to check your diet and physical activity. Therefore, it simplifies and personalizes the process of diet monitoring for a lot of people who cannot afford personal experts to be at their beck and call.

Chapter Twelve:
Final Goals of Carb Cycling

Most of the diets that exist are made up of placing protein as the central macronutrient. What separates carb cycling with other dieting strategies is its ability to value all macronutrients and make use of them to regulate lifestyles.

While it is essential to understand the details of our diets, it is equally vital to recall that our minds and bodies are intimately interconnected. Health is as psychological as it is physical. Most foods that aim at making our body devoid of essential nutrients have an adverse impact on our psychology. Therefore, it is important to remember at all points in time that carb cycling or any other dieting strategy is a holistic process. It couples nutrient fluctuation with physical activity to generate a wholesome body.

In the strategy of carb cycling, one nutrient is the variable, in this case, carbohydrate, and the others are always fixed. Fluctuation never occurs in proteins or fats, and it must be limited to carbohydrates to achieve proper results. This focus on incorporating all nutrients is one that ensures nutrient diversity in the body that fulfills all the various needs we exist with.

There are certain specific aspects of carb cycling we must revisit in order to completely link together the strategy and the philosophy of carb cycling.

Carb cycling is a strategy where carbohydrates are the variable. At first glance it seems like a heavy prioritization of carbs as the central macronutrient. The underlying nuance we often misconstrue is that the diet strategy aids in the essential macronutrients that are kept fixed for optimum utilization. Protein is a macronutrient that forms our life force. It is important to understand its general significance to grasp the carb fluctuation formula of the strategy.

To link all the practical directions of carb cycling to its scientific basis, it is important to delve into the theory of macronutrient regulation in humans.

The three central macronutrients are carbohydrates, proteins, and fats.

The behavioral naturalness of feeding and appetite regulation are critical processes for survival. It is providing the body with the proper amount of macro and micronutrients happens through appetite regulation of proper quantities of fat, protein, and carbohydrates. The strategy of regulating a select macronutrient is a feature not merely unique to man but is observed in rodents as well. There is a genetic selection of macronutrient preference in a scenario where the species are dependent on the process of diurnal variation. This occurs through processes of pre-ingestive signals and post-ingestive signals.

How does one then apply this scientific jargon to everyday life?

Through our discussion of carb cycling and the many guidelines that come with it, we have achieved the conclusion that the body is a system that functions on certain essential nutrients for survival. In a scenario where we want the body to change its response strategy for alterations of physique or internal health, it needs to be made adept to a certain kind of consumption pattern. The process of carb cycling is a strictly regulated diet plan that aims at manipulating the consumption of carbs while keeping all other macronutrients stagnant. This is labeled as a process of body hacking, as discussed in earlier chapters.

The major reasons for the health problems that people experience comes from the inconsistency of macronutrient consumption. The way carb cycling solves this problem is by reorienting the body into balanced nutrient consumption through a combination of dietary practices and physical activity. Therefore, it succeeds in solving the problem of both lack and excess consumption.

There are certain guidelines you need to follow in order to gain the maximum benefits of carb cycling, as discussed below.

Mitigating Side Effects

There are diets that aim at a straightforward reduction of carbohydrates. Compared to such a diet, carb cycling allows for imagining a diet that is balanced and can be maintained easily without the weight of dietary restrictions.

The importance of exercise needs to be reiterated. On a high carb day, its alignment with exercise enables the extra calories derived from carbohydrates and nutrients associated with it to help utilize energy to bring out intensity.

This paves the way for you to make the most of your training.

At a time where research is dominated by the benefits of a low carb diet, and an absence of the scientific impacts specific to carb cycling, the difference needs to be explicitly stated.

The central difference between a low carb diet and carb cycling would be the stagnant state of less carb intake where the diet constitutes of all low carb days in contrast to adhering to a fluctuating low carb state as followed in carb cycling. There is a restriction of carbs in both scenarios, with the common fact remaining that low carbs cause weight loss.

Since it is important to combine carb cycling with training, its unique benefit is the proper supply of carbs on training days. In case there is a deficiency of carbs while exercising, as in a stagnant low carb diet, healthy performance is hindered. There are many physiological benefits experienced by athletes who follow carb cycling.

This is attributed to the fact that carbohydrates are the main energy resources for fuelling the ability to undergo high-intensity exercises. It builds endurance since it mitigates the feeling of weakness that comes from carb deficiency caused by a low carb diet. Therefore, it builds endurance and helps to fight fatigue.

Therefore, the central benefit of the carb cycling diet is its ability to fuel physical activity. This makes it not only a practical diet but also one that encourages you to combine the two central notions of health, exercise and healthy eating.

The side effects of carb cycling probably manifest from the inclusion of lower carb days as it makes the individual undergoing the diet susceptible to feelings of lethargy and hunger. This is due to the accidental neglect of the consumption of essential nutrients such as fiber.

However, the principle of flexibility, which is distinct from carb cycling helps to solve this problem. Due to this it's a process of constantly switching from lower carb days to medium carb days to high carb days and vice versa. The downsides of this are mitigated almost completely.

The Principle of Flexibility

The central principle of carb cycling is the idea of flexibility. It recognizes that a diet alone cannot cause changes in your body. It stresses on letting the diet be adjusted according to the context that helps you maintain a balance.

No matter what diet we consider, the restriction of calories always causes the metabolic rate to slow down considerably. It also has an impact on hormones that are responsible for causing the sensation of hunger. Therefore, making anyone following this diet susceptible to weight regain. According to research, to raise metabolism temporarily, carb loading can be helpful. While also increasing levels of leptin in the body at the same time, which is a hormone that suppresses hunger. All this combined together could aid in weight loss.

As mentioned earlier, carbohydrate-laden foods are the powerhouse for the athletic body as they boost an athlete's performance, endurance and recovery. The science behind has got to do with the ability of carbohydrate-based fuel sources getting burned for generating energy. Protein is spared and is utilized for muscle growth and not wasted as fuel.

Common thinking talks about the idea that high carb days once in a blue moon can aid non-athletes in the prevention of their metabolism from slowing down. It can raise the effectiveness of their workouts, aid in weight reduction, and help to build muscle while low carb days could be dedicated to helping the body burn all the fat accumulation as fuel.

Before we approach carb cycling, we need to ingrain in our mind that there is no proven scientific formula to it. You must, therefore, keep an open mind and be open to hectic alteration in your diet and lifestyle plans.

During the course of the carb cycle, it must be noted that hitting specific calorie goals to shed weight or to build muscle remains an important aspect. The focus should be on wholesome, healthy, and good quality whole foods. The nature of carbs incorporated in your diet can have a great impact on your health.

For instance, consuming refined carbs will not aid in any benefits. For carb cycling to work, one must stick to the consumption of good carbs. A further example of this would be the consumption of products with added sugar, such as soda and candy, or food consisting of starch like white bread and white rice. It must be reiterated that they aren't health-conscious choices. You must pick carbohydrates profuse with nutrients that remain low on the glycemic index. Examples of these would be quinoa, beans, oats, and sweet potatoes.

Another guideline that you must follow is to remember not to overeat on high carb days. The central distinction between high carb days and low carb days is not as wide as you may imagine. A high carb day should not be confused for a "cheat day" when you can eat whatever you wish.

The benefit of carb cycling is that it's much easier to stick to its flexible methods over time as compared to a low carb diet. Health is beyond weight loss and rigorous training, and such a strategy offers a way out for people who do not want to indulge in either. The idea is to promote a gradual reduction in refined carbs, which cause obesity and other problems. This will promote fat reduction for some individuals.

However, the fact remains that there isn't enough scientific literature on carb cycling diet yet to make a legitimate claim about its exact effects.

The one way in which you can make full use of this, however, is by following the principle of consistency. To get results, you must pick the proper kind of carbohydrates in proper quantities. This ensures a healthy eating pattern, which is very directly linked to the prevention of lethal diseases like cancer, stroke, and heart disease.

Even if you cannot focus on the exact grams or percentages of macronutrients such as carbs, fats, and proteins, you could replace some of the unhealthy food you consume by whole foods. Examples of these would include fish, fruit, poultry, seeds, beans, nuts, vegetables, and whole grains.

The best kind of diet plan that you can follow is one that is based on the principle of sustainability. While carb cycling does rely on calculations and accurate proportions to get results, the nature of its flexibility ensures that it can be customized according to the person taking up the diet completely.

Experimentation is key is when it comes to approaching carb cycling.

Each person is a unique individual with a distinct body type that functions on different needs. It is fallacious to assume that one kind of formula can work for everyone in the same way. The people indulging in the strategy of carb cycling have different motives and agendas. To be satisfied and healthy, you must approach a dietician at the earliest.

One piece of advice that must be repeated is the importance of professional help to aid lifestyle changes. Food consumption is often not seen seriously enough by individuals.

You'll be surprised to know that the worst side effect of a consistent low carb diet could be a threat to your life. Therefore, management of macronutrients in the most balanced way possible must be ensured at every step of the way. The combination of different consumption days does this job by making sure you do not calcify into an unhealthy pattern of behavior.

Therefore, do not hesitate to go ahead and give healthy living a try and redefine what dieting means to you.

Conclusion

At the end of this book, I would like to thank everyone who took the time to read it. I hope that your interest in carb cycling and its merits have been sufficiently piqued. If you were already interested in the method, I hope that you have acquired enough knowledge to apply carb cycling to your life. If you do so, I hope this book is a handy manual and your one-stop guide for all carb cycling related queries.

Carb cycling, in conclusion, is a high-level, yet simple method that can be customized to suit anyone's needs and goals. It is a method that works on the whole body, internally and externally. Moreover, it encourages a lifestyle of calorie counting and monitoring your body. Limitless variations of carb cycling are possible, but if you follow the basic cycling principle, you will lose weight and gain muscle gradually.

You need to commit to the golden rule of eating healthy and pick your carbohydrates wisely. A detailed breakdown of how to know which carbs are good for you has been given in the book, along with many examples that specify certain good carbohydrates.

If you follow all the detailed plans and tips given in this book, you will notice the changes in your body.

Carb cycling produces many healthy changes within your body. You must keep monitoring your progress using the tools mentioned in this book. Create a chart of the calories you consume, and start documenting every low, high, and medium carb day. You can get your dream body, and feel the comfort of living healthily.

Do not lose hope if the changes are not physically visible in the first few days of the diet. Using the methods outlined in this book, you will be able to fix the imbalance of nutrients within your body. This will gradually lead to the physical changes that you desire.

Always remember that a healthy mind produces a healthy body. Nourish your mind with a balanced diet and positive thoughts. Get in touch with nature by exercising outdoors. Physical fitness is always a combination of good food and regular exercise.

Make sure you use this diet to get in touch with your inner self. Honor your body like the majestic creation it is by feeding it nutritious fruits and vegetables. The meal plans mentioned in this book will aid you in having fun in your dieting journey.

If you follow all the detailed plans and suggestions given in this book, you will notice the transformation in your body.

There are many diets out there, but carb cycling is the most scientific and accessible high-level diet of them all. It is bound to get you back in touch with your body and make you truly become aware of what it requires.

You will find yourself treating your body with a lot of care and giving it only that which will make it stronger.

THE END... almost!

Reviews are vital in spreading the word about books. However, they are not easy to come by.

As an independent author with a tiny marketing budget, I rely on readers, like you, to leave a short review on Amazon.

Even if it is just a sentence or two!

So if you enjoyed the book, please leave a brief review on Amazon.

I am very appreciative for your review as it truly makes a difference.

Thank you from the bottom of my heart for purchasing this book and reading it to the end!

Yours sincerely, fellow companion in exiting journey to the best shape in your life
John Carver

References

3 body types, how to work and eat for them! (From the Blog of Heart Core Fitness Studio of Cape Cod). (2019). Retrieved from http://heartcorestudio.com/blog/entry/3-body-types-how-to-work-and-eat-for-them

Andrews, R. All About Carb Cycling | Precision Nutrition. Retrieved from https://www.precisionnutrition.com/all-about-carb-cycling

Carb Cycling: The 30-Day Nutrition Plan That Actually Works. (2019). Retrieved from https://www.mymetabolicmeals.com/carb-cycling-the-30-day-nutrition-plan-that-actually-works/

Henry, A. (2013). Retrieved from https://lifehacker.com/five-best-food-and-nutrition-tracking-tools-1084103754

Iliades, C. (2010). The Importance of Water in Your Diet Plan. Retrieved from https://www.everydayhealth.com/weight/the-importance-of-water-in-your-diet-plan.aspx

Mawer, R. (2017). What is Carb Cycling and How Does it Work?. Retrieved from https://www.healthline.com/nutrition/carb-cycling-101

Matthews, M. (2019). The Science of Carb Cycling: How It Works and How to Do It Right (2019). Retrieved from https://legionathletics.com/carb-cycling/

Monitoring nutrition: the national diet and nutrition survey. (2019). Retrieved from https://www.futurelearn.com/courses/musculoskeletal/0/steps/25173

Sharp, A. (2017). Carb Cycling: Should You Be Carbohydrate Cycling to Lose Weight?. Retrieved from https://www.abbeyskitchen.com/carb-cycling/

What is metabolism?. (2015). Retrieved from https://www.healio.com/endocrinology/news/online/%7Be28 2a7f3-47a1-43a5-96bf-71a6d545e4ee%7D/what-is-metabolism

What Are Nutrients?. (2019). Retrieved from https://med.libretexts.org/Courses/Sacramento_City_College /SCC%3A_Nutri_300_(Coppola)/Text/01%3A_Nutrition_an d_You/1.2%3A_What_Are_Nutrients%3F

Whiteman, H. (2019). The effects of aging: can they be reversed?. Retrieved from https://www.medicalnewstoday.com/articles/307383.php

Carb Cycling Lifestyle for Women

Women

A Painless Diet Plan to Lose Weight and Enjoy Your Life

John Carver

Table of Contents

Introduction

Weight loss might still be an incredibly sensitive and taboo topic for a lot of people. These days, you have to be very careful when you talk about a person's weight because you never know when you might offend someone. However, in spite of that, more and more people are starting to adopt healthier lifestyles and are more open to discussing the harsh realities of getting fit and healthy. Because the truth is that while we picture fit and healthy people as always so happy and positive, the road to getting fit is not a glamorous one. It's harsh. It's a struggle. And unfortunately, this is the reason why a lot of people just end up quitting a short time after they begin. They realize that their expectations were false to begin with, and they become disappointed when their results are not up to par.

This book is going to help you manage your expectations better so that you not only go into your weight loss journey with the right approach, but you also go into it with the right mindset. Remember that mindset makes up a huge part of the game. You need to have the proper disposition going into any difficult endeavor if you are hoping to find success in it. Of course, more than just telling you what to do to be healthier, this book is also going to orient you on the many things that you need to prepare your mind for to tackle this problem. And make no mistake about it, obesity really is a problem.

People shouldn't have to be shamed by others for wanting to lose weight. It's the same as when someone enrolls in school to learn about a new academic field or when someone takes up a new hobby to master a new craft. People who go on diets or undergo physical exercise regimens are just people who are seeking to make their lives better. They understand that there is a problem with the way that they are living their lives and that there is room for improvement. And don't doubt the fact that so many people in the world have problems with their weight.

According to data that was published in *The Lancet* journal, more than 3.4 million human deaths worldwide were caused by overweight- or obesity-related diseases in 2014 (Afshin et al., 2019). The same data set that was published in the article revealed that there have been 27.5% and 47.1% upticks in the number of overweight and obese adults and children respectively since 1980. Those are alarming numbers and the statistics don't make for very good future prospects in health and fitness. Obesity is a very serious public health issue that needs to be addressed on both a policy level and a personal level. According to the World Obesity Federation, more than $850 billion is spent per year on direct healthcare costs for people who are obese or overweight (World Economic Forum, 2018). So, obesity isn't just a matter of compromising one's physical health. It's also compromising peoples' financial well-being as well.

However, as echoed in an article published by the World Economic Forum, the common sentiment is not that people don't have the willpower or the conviction to want to be healthy (Ryan, Candeias, & Jorgensen, 2018). A lot of the blame regarding why obesity persists in being a global problem today rests on the fact that there are still a lot of misinformation and outdated perceptions on health and wellness. All of these conflicting data and ideas have accounted for people to lead very unhealthy lives even though they believe they are doing the opposite. This is why there is a need to further push for more science-backed recommendations on how to tackle weight loss and obesity.

Hence, this book.

Of course, there are a myriad of literary sources out there that are available for your consumption. Why should you trust this one in particular? We've already talked about how in this age of information, there are certain dangers surrounding misinformation and the peddling of fake news. Naturally, you should be skeptical of everything that you read, right? That's only natural. No one would blame you for wanting to authenticate everything that you read, especially when it concerns your health and well-being.

So, in an attempt to assuage your apprehensions and skepticism, perhaps it would be a good idea for you to get to know the person behind the words that you're currently reading.

About the Author

John Carver is a health expert and author who was born and raised on the island of Bermuda. He completed his tertiary studies at university in Washington, DC, and took his professional practice to California where he got a job for a prominent retail company. It was during this early stage of his career wherein he really dedicated himself to the realms of health and fitness. He embarked on a very vigorous training and exercise program as he set bigger and higher goals for himself.

However, it was only after a friend had given him insights into how his diet was affecting his physical performance during training when John quickly realized that his approach was lacking in something vital. He discovered that he also needed to be paying just as much attention to the food that he was eating as well. It wasn't just about the effort that he was putting into his training sessions. It was also about the fuel and the nutrients that he was putting into his body. This is when John decided that he needed to change his outlook and take a new approach to his fitness.

A new enterprise—selling health supplements—along with an enhanced training regimen, meant that John took much greater care of what he ate and in particular of the carbohydrates he consumed. That, in turn, led to much better performances in the competitions he entered, but the biggest change came when he decided to spread his knowledge and share his experiences to a wider audience.

His book, *Carb Cycling: The Science and Practice of Mastering Your Metabolism*, has proven to be an exciting addition to books that not only help athletes look after their bodies, but also provide help for people who are keen to lose weight and take care of themselves better. Of course, the dietary needs of different people are going to differ based on the kinds of lives that they lead. This is a point that John has stressed in depth in his books. However, through his guidance and education, plenty of people, regardless of fitness backgrounds or athletic levels, have managed to find success in their own personal fitness goals.

Given the impact that he has made on countless lives, John is planning other books along the same lines and is embarking on expanding his business further. He hopes that by doing so, he will reach out to even more people who will reap the same rewards that he has.

In his spare time, John enjoys running, cooking, and spending lots of time with his girlfriend. He loves nothing better than spending days at the beach, grilling food on an open fire, and watching the stars with an occasional cold beer and great friends around him.

A Fitness Movement for Women

Again, it's important to emphasize the fact that different people are going to have different needs and prescriptions when it comes to their fitness activities or dietary practices. This is why this book isn't going to be in the business of providing any cookie-cutter advice that is aimed at a general audience. The information and advice that will be listed here should be fit for women, in particular, who are looking to get healthier and fitter through carb cycling.

When it comes to health and wellness, one must always consider the fact that certain practices are only effective depending on the physiological responses of the human body. And given that men and women have very different physical makeups, it's important to emphasize that the approaches to health and fitness for each gender are more specialized and streamlined relative to the ways that their bodies are constructed. This book goes the extra mile by providing some very key insights into how women's bodies are constructed and how they adapt to certain fitness and dietary programs. You must realize that achieving health and wellness is a very nuanced endeavor and that there are many nuances to dieting and exercising. It can be very overwhelming to have to gather, absorb, and practice all of these nuances that come from scattered sources. This is why this book is going to curate all of the information and knowledge that you need to know in order for you to really find success in your health and wellness goals.

The road to achieving optimal health and wellness is not an easy one. And it definitely isn't one that guarantees immediate success either. It's a lot of ups and downs, rises and falls, highs and lows. Sure, you might find success in the initial phases of it, but you shouldn't expect your success to be consistent or linear. Expect a lot of speed bumps, setbacks, and major hurdles in this journey of yours. However, you shouldn't fret.

It's important that you understand the value of embracing the process. As early as now, you need to develop the conviction that is necessary to carry you through the tough journey that you're going to take. It's definitely not going to be without its fair share of difficulties. But nothing worth having in life ever comes easily anyway.

You shouldn't let the difficulty or enormity of the challenge that faces you be intimidating enough to make you want to give up. This is why this book and many others like it exist. This book is going to guide you through every step of the way. Remember that whenever you are faced with a wall that you feel like you can't overcome, someone else has stood exactly where you are right now. And that same person has managed to overcome that wall to keep on pushing through. If it can work for them, then it should also work for you.

Carb cycling is a scientifically proven and trusted method for losing weight and getting healthier. Not only that, it has also managed to help athletes all over the world improve their athletic performance significantly. These improvements have led them to break through walls and barriers that were previously impervious to their efforts. Sure, you can always lose a few pounds here and there by exercising really hard and committing to a strict training regimen. But if you don't have a diet that is able to properly nourish you and supplement your workouts, then you won't really be able to maximize your potential.

So, this is why one must always need to take a holistic and well-rounded approach to getting fit. You can't be a great exerciser without paying attention to the food that you eat. And you can't be a healthy eater if you're just going to end up not using any of your calories and sitting around all day. Diet and exercise are two things that go hand-in-hand. And there are all sorts of diet and exercise programs out there that many people have found success in. However, for the woman who is looking for an effective and sustainable way of achieving all her health and wellness goals, there is carb cycling. If you are ready to take a deep dive into the world of carb cycling, then let's journey into the first chapter of this book together.

Chapter 1:
Welcome to Carb Cycling

If you're a parent, you would never allow your small child to dive into a pool without knowing how deep it is first, right? When you're sick, you never want to take any medicine without first understanding how it's going to affect your body. When you see a nice pair of expensive shoes at a designer store that you're interested in, you want to find out everything you need to know about that shoe before you pour a lot of money into buying it. This is the same kind of approach that anyone should take to adopting a new diet or exercise routine. You don't want to dive into carb cycling without first understanding the principles behind it. You should always orient and familiarize yourself first with all that there is to know about carb cycling so that you are tackling and approaching it the right way.

Of course, it's not just about ensuring your own safety and wellness. Sure, there are certain diets out there that might prove to be effective for certain types of people but can be just as dangerous for others. For example, a high-protein or high-fat diet might not exactly be ideal for a patient with kidney disease even though these tend to be very popular "weight loss" diets for most other people. A Mediterranean diet, which is high in carbs, isn't going to be the best one for patients who are diabetic or who have high blood sugar levels. However, there are plenty of others who will swear that adopting the Mediterranean diet has helped them become fitter and healthier. Again, it all depends on the person and how their body responds to a certain diet.

Prior to trying out carb cycling, you first have to determine if it's the right diet for you. And the first step to doing so is making sure that you understand all of the key information and details surrounding carb cycling. From there, you will have a more refined and insightful opinion on the matter.

However, more than just knowing if it would be a safe and plausible diet for you, it's important that you approach the diet the right way. You will never be able to find success in any endeavor if you don't take the time to properly familiarize and orient yourself with it first. There are plenty of novices out there who only read the headlines surrounding certain diet fads without acquainting themselves with the fine print. They end up approaching the diet the wrong way, and they don't get the results that were promised to them. You never want to fall into the same kind of trap. A huge part of finding success in a difficult endeavor such as this is making sure that you have all bases covered with regards to your approach to it.

This is exactly what this chapter is going to try to help you out with. If you're coming from a place where you know absolutely nothing about carb cycling, then there's no need to worry. By the time you finish reading this chapter, you will be in a much better position than before. You will be briefed on the idea of carb cycling and how it impacts your body to help stimulate weight loss and improved athletic performance. You will also be exposed to the science behind carb cycling and why it works for so many people. Don't worry. You don't need a degree in nutrition or biomechanics to understand the science behind it. This chapter is also going to delve deeper into the effectiveness of carb cycling relative to other similar diet styles.

All of this information is valuable knowledge that will allow you to determine whether this is the diet for you. This knowledge is also going to help you on your path should you proceed to go this route towards health and fitness. Now, this prompts us to ask the question, what exactly is carb cycling?

What Is Carb Cycling and How Do You Do It?

Carbs have been demonized by the health and fitness community for the longest time now. You probably hear about it all the time. *Lay off the carbs. Cut out the sugar. Stop eating donuts.* Carbs have really gotten a bad rep in the dieting world. But is all that hate really warranted? There are all sorts of popular diet programs out there that dramatically restrict carbohydrate consumption. Heck, there are even certain diets out there that get rid of carbs altogether. Are carbs really all that bad?

Just in case you don't already know, carbs actually comprise just one of the three macronutrients that should be making up your daily diet. The other macronutrients are proteins and fats. Given that, it's important to emphasize that there is no one macronutrient that is inherently unhealthy or bad. All macronutrients, or *macros,* have their place in the nourishment of the human body. These macros all serve very distinct and specific purposes. It's only when humans overindulge or abuse the consumption of certain macros that it becomes bad and unhealthy.

Essentially, the carb cycling diet program is based on the principle that carbohydrates don't necessarily have to be restricted per se. The consumption of carbs under carb cycling just has to be managed and tailored properly relative to the needs of the individual. To be more concrete about it, people who go through carb cycling just alternate the intervals wherein they maximize and minimize their carb consumptions.

The durations of these intervals can vary depending on the individual. Some people cycle through their carbs on a daily, weekly, biweekly, or even monthly basis. Ultimately, the whole point of carb cycling is to stimulate fat burn while also improving athletic performance in spite of caloric restrictions. At the same time, carb cycling is a sustainable means of tackling weight loss plateaus. Typically, people who go on diets and don't change things up after sustained success are bound to hit a weight loss plateau. Essentially, a plateau takes place whenever the body adapts or acclimates itself to the dietary habits of an individual to the point where it starts burning less fat in an effort to retain more fat reserves. This is just the body's natural response to make sure that there is a lot of stored energy left in the body in case of emergencies. Of course, if you are looking to sustain weight loss for the long term, you need to break through these plateaus. And this is where carb cycling can be very effective.

Again, keep in mind that carbohydrates are not inherently bad. All macros serve a very distinct and specific purpose. However, what the carb cycling method does is minimize one's chances of consuming carbohydrates in excess and during times when they don't really need it. Through a popular carb cycling program, one would only consume carbohydrates during moments when they provide maximum benefits and in the proper degrees. There are a variety of factors that can influence the manner in which you might structure your carb cycling program. Here are just some of them:

Current Body Mass/Fat Levels

For the casual person who is trying to lose weight, they only need to look at the current state of their bodies. Again, it's going to differ depending on how your body is currently structured. However, the general rule of thumb here is that the leaner you are, then the higher number of high-carb consumption intervals or blocks you would have.

Body Mass/Composition Goals

This is a variable that factors in greatly to those who are really looking to chisel their physiques to the greatest level of detail. This carb cycling variable is most important to bodybuilders who are training for competitions or events. Essentially, they divide their carb cycling into phases depending on where they are in their training regimen. For mass bulking and bodybuilding, one would increase carb consumption. And for mass cutting, one would minimize carb consumption as much as possible.

Training Schedule

Another big factor that most people consider when plotting out their carb cycling intervals is the training schedule. One general principle that people follow is that they maximize carb consumption on training days, and they minimize carb consumption on rest days. The principle behind this is that the body doesn't need as many carbohydrates to function and perform properly when it isn't put through a strenuous workout. So, it would be best to minimize carb consumption during these days.

Training Intensity

Sometimes, it's not just a matter of consuming large amounts of carbohydrates on training days and restricting carbs on rest days. Some athletes will really go into detail by factoring in the level of intensity that they exert during workouts on certain days. However, the principles of carb cycling still remain consistent. The more intense or more physically demanding a training session is, then the higher the demand for carbohydrates on that day. Conversely, when training sessions are light and relatively easy, then the lower the requirements for carbs.

Fitness Events/Competitions

This variable of carb cycling might be just for a select group of people but it's still worth mentioning. There are certain athletes out there who just aren't training to be fit or healthy. There are athletes who are training towards competitions or sporting events. Sometimes, they will structure their carb cycling patterns based on the schedule of their competitions and events. Some athletes might overindulge on carbs in the lead-up to endurance-based events like marathons or triathlons. Some athletes might cut out carbs in the lead-up to certain events like bodybuilding competitions or photo shoots.

What Makes Carb Cycling So Effective?

Sure, now you may get the basic gist of what carb cycling is and how people incorporate it into their daily lives. Now, we ask the question: how does it work? Earlier, we discussed how carb cycling is a dietary pattern that is proven to be effective for many different people who have differing goals. If you're someone who is trying to train for an athletic competition, carb cycling can help fuel your athletic performance. If you're someone who has to lose some weight quickly for a special event, carb cycling can help you get the job done. Even if you're just someone who wants to stay trim and healthy over a sustainable period, carb cycling can help you out with that as well.

It seems too good to be true that a simple carb consumption pattern can impact so many kinds of people with different goals in a positive manner. However, it shouldn't be too difficult to believe in the carb cycling philosophy once you take the time to understand the science behind it and how it affects your body.

The Science Behind Carb Cycling

Compared to other mainstream dietary programs and philosophies, carb cycling is relatively new. This means that the scientific data surrounding carb cycling may not be as exhaustive as compared to those of diets like keto or Paleo. However, as you continue to read on, you will learn that the evidence is actually compelling enough to make a solid case for itself in terms of effectiveness and sustainability. Essentially, all of the scientific principles surrounding carb cycling have to do with the natural bodily reactions that are associated with the manipulation of carbohydrate consumption.

Before you can understand the science behind carb cycling,

you must first understand what carbs are and why the body needs them in the first place. Essentially, in order for your body to function properly, it needs energy. Your body gets this energy from glucose. The glucose that your body converts into energy comes from the calories that you consume on a daily basis. Your calories stem mostly from your macronutrients that we have already discussed earlier: protein, fat, and carbohydrates. However, the macronutrient that has the most efficient properties for glucose conversion is carbs. So, this is why a lot of people tend to associate carbohydrates with energy. When the body is deprived of calories to convert into glucose, it targets the reserves (the body's accumulated fats) and converts those into glucose for energy instead.

So, with that in mind, this is where carb cycling comes in. Ideally, when plotting a carb cycling program, one would manipulate carb consumption levels relative to the demands of the body. When the body doesn't need too much energy to perform or function adequately, then carb consumption must be managed to meet those needs and not exceed them. The reason that carbs should ideally be limited on nonintense days (or rest days) is because the body doesn't really need to expend much energy to function properly. Hence, any excess carbohydrates or glucose might end up getting converted to stored fat instead. This could be problematic for anyone whose goals are to get leaner and trimmer, especially around the waist.

However, it's not just about losing weight. Again, athletes who care about their physical performance may also engage in carb cycling. This is where high-carb days during the carb cycling program come in. Usually, when workouts get really strenuous, athletes will struggle with recovery and rejuvenation to sustain a long-term training plan. Consuming large amounts of carbohydrates can aid in refueling the glycogen in muscles. This means that muscles aren't broken down so much and are quicker at recovering for more workouts.

There is also another layer to the carb cycling method, and it has something to do with hormone manipulation in the body. Leptin and ghrelin are hormones that regulate a person's weight and appetite and that are produced within the body. Through strategic carb cycling, the production of these hormones is regulated optimally so as to stimulate fat burn while also suppressing unnecessary hunger pangs.

During low-carb days, the body is sometimes forced to enter a carb-fasted state. At its most extreme form, this is sometimes referred to as ketosis wherein the body's liver produces ketones which serve as the replacements for glucose that comes from carbohydrates. In order to produce ketones, the body has to burn off stored fat in the body. This is where fat loss is at its most optimal. Instead of relying on the calories that one consumes for energy, the body tries to become more self-sustaining by burning off more of its reserves instead. However, low-carb consumption days on a carb cycling diet don't really call for one to enter a state of ketosis. Those are only requirements of a keto diet. But more on that later. Ultimately, it is said that carb cycling can help stimulate the body's metabolism and burn fat at a more efficient rate.

Lastly, the final scientific layer to the effectiveness of carb cycling has to do with insulin sensitivity. Essentially, by strategically minimizing or cutting out carbs from a diet, the body's insulin levels are regulated properly so as not to induce weight gain, diabetes, or heart disease.

The Difference Between Carb Cycling and Keto

If you've already done your research about dieting and fitness prior to reading this book, then there is a very good chance that you've already encountered the idea of keto. It was already previously mentioned in this chapter that keto is a dietary form of restricting one's self from consuming carbohydrates so as to induce a state of ketosis in the body (or a ketogenic state). So, if keto is also a diet that promotes the minimal consumption of carbohydrates, then what makes it less or more effective than carb cycling? If carb cycling is the restriction of carb intake through intervals, wouldn't a stagnant state of restriction result in better outcomes for weight loss? These are some very valid questions, and it's definitely okay for you to be asking them. But before we get to the root of the answer, we need to dig deeper beyond the surface levels of each dietary proposition.

A Deep Dive Into Ketosis

Think of your body as a machine that runs on fuel. This fuel can come in many different forms through the food that you eat. However, your body as a machine has a natural personal preference in where it sources its fuel. For the most part, it chooses to process carbs over the other two macronutrients. The reason for that is because carbs are the easiest for the body to process into glucose, which is used to energize your body and keep the machine running operationally.

So, as has already been explained earlier, the carbs that you eat get processed into its simplest form, called glucose. This glucose is then picked up and pushed through your bloodstream to distribute energy all throughout your body. However, not all of this glucose is used up by your body, especially on days when you're not being physically active. This is when your glucose ends up getting stored as fat.

141

Getting Fat From Carbs

Once your body has determined that all of your caloric needs are met, whatever glucose is left behind doesn't get used up and is stored in the body's reserves. So, if we go back to the analogy of the machine, when you're taking in too much glucose, you are going to start overflowing with fuel. All of that excess energy has to go somewhere. Naturally, what the body does is it converts all of that unused glucose into stored energy called glycogen.

Later on, when your body starts running out of energy, it takes whatever stored glycogen is left and converts it back into glucose to fuel the body. Over time, if the glycogen really doesn't get used up, it turns into the visible fat that you see on your arms, waist, legs, and the rest of your body. This is why you end up getting those love handles whenever you aren't burning off more than you're eating.

Why Ketosis is Good for Weight Loss

So, given all of that information surrounding the processing of carbohydrates, simple logic will tell you that the key to losing weight would be to make sure that you're burning off more energy than you're eating. However, what ketosis does is take the fat-burning process a step further by forcing the body to burn its own reserved fats instead of the energy that you're eating through your food. Again, as has been previously mentioned, this fat-burning process by carb restriction is called putting your body into a ketogenic state.

The way that the keto diet works is that it always pushes for your body to be in a perpetual state of ketosis. This way, your body is constantly trying to burn off its reserved fats in order to sustain itself. Originally, ketosis was actually an experiment that was used to treat patients who were experiencing seizures or epilepsy. There was evidence that suggested that ketogenic patients had better experiences when dealing with seizures. However, it has mostly evolved to become a weight loss tool, especially in this modern age.

Keto vs. Carb Cycling: Which Is better?

So, to sum it all up, keto is essentially the perpetual restriction or minimization of carbohydrate consumption to induce a constant state of ketosis in the body to stimulate one's metabolism. This is why a lot of people tend to adopt the keto diet whenever they're trying to meet specific weight loss goals such as reaching a target weight on the scale or being able to fit into an old pair of jeans.

On the other hand, there is carb cycling. This is a dietary philosophy that encourages intervals of high-carb and low-carb consumption days. If you take away the component of intervals in carb cycling, it should share a lot of the same principles as the keto diet. However, there is a substantial difference in terms of execution and results. As you are plotting your carb cycling routine, you would never really aim to induce a state of ketosis in your body, not even on your low-carb days. Ketosis is not a requirement for traditional carb cycling. Also, the main difference between keto and carb cycling is the duration of carb restriction. With keto, it's a perpetual state of restriction. With carb cycling, the durations for restriction are strategically timed.

Now, it's time for us to answer the question: which one is better?

You might hate this answer, but the truth is that it depends. It really depends on the kind of goals that you have and what kind of personality you have as well. At the end of the day, it's all about being able to find a diet that works for you. Sustainability is key here. Sure, you might find immediate success with a keto diet, but would you really be able to sustain carb restrictions for the long term? Of course, you might find comfort in the carb cycling diet, but will it be able to provide you with the results that you want in the time that you set for yourself? It's all relative. Again, it all boils down to whatever works best for you. And while that may be the safe and unsatisfying answer, it's also what is true.

The Middle Ground: Keto Cycling

For those who want to marry both dieting principles, there is also such a thing as keto cycling. And it's exactly what it sounds like. Essentially, you would induce a state of ketosis in your body, but you would only do so in intervals. So, like the carb cycling scheduling format, you would have keto days and nonketo days. For a lot of people who want to reap the dramatic benefits of ketosis, this is a more sustainable way of going about it as it doesn't completely eliminate carbohydrate consumption altogether.

However, that isn't the only variable that you want to take into consideration when deciding for yourself what dietary program to undertake. There are certain pros and cons that are attached to each dietary principle which will make them more distinct. It would be best for you to gather more information about keto, carb cycling, keto cycling, and any other dietary program before you come to a decision. Again, knowledge is power.

The Highs and Lows of Carb Cycling

Ultimately, getting into a carb cycling diet just means having high carb and low carb days. The key is in making sure that all of the numbers add up and that you're distributing your high- and low-carb days properly. Again, there are a variety of factors that you need to consider when determining when your high- and low-carb days are going to be. You have to consider your current body mass composition, target body composition, training schedule, training intensity, etc. However, the general idea here is that you don't go too many consecutive days of just having either high- or low-carb consumption. You want to mix it up as much as possible.

High-Carb Days

Again, the numbers can vary from person to person. However, if you're just starting out, you won't want to stray too far away from the recommended number of 60% of calories consumed from carbohydrates. So, if you're eating 2,000 calories a day, that means you should be eating 1,200 calories from carbohydrates during high-carb days. As you gain more experience and practice in carb cycling, you can tweak the numbers to meet your specific needs as you go.

It's also important to really listen to your body when you're engaged in a strict training regimen. If you feel like you're feeling gassed just 5 minutes into a workout, it might be due to you not having enough carbs to work with. Sometimes, not having enough carbs can also translate to you feeling groggy or tired when you're at the office, and you're unable to focus on your work.

However, it's very important that you don't have a "treat yourself" mindset when determining your high-carb consumption numbers. It's very dangerous to think "I ran an extra mile today, so I get to have an extra 50g of carbs." If you have a plan, try to stick to it as much as possible. You shouldn't be in the business of rewarding yourself with food. You should merely see the food that you eat as a source of nourishment for your body. It shouldn't be a prize that you get for being disciplined. Otherwise, you would be defeating the purpose of going on a diet.

Low-Carb Days

Typically, you would want to schedule your low-carb days on those days where you aren't really expending too much energy. So, perhaps on days when you're just doing less intense exercises like light jogging, yoga, or even when you're just taking a rest from working out altogether, it would be best for you to not overindulge in carbs. So, during high-carb days, you would typically load up on complex carbohydrates that come from wheats, starches, and other similar sources. On low-carb days, you will want to exchange those complex carbs for some leafy greens, lean meats, and healthy fats like oils or nuts.

To be more concrete about it, take this as an example. During high-carb days, you might have a turkey burger on a whole-wheat bun for dinner. This would be fine on a high-carb day. However, on a low-carb day, you can take this same meal and replace the whole-wheat bun with lettuce, tomatoes, onions, low-carb dressing, and even cheese.

Shifting Cycles

One of the best parts about going on a carb cycling program is that your body has a difficult time acclimating itself to what you're doing. A lot of the time, when people just completely restrict themselves from eating for prolonged periods, their bodies adapt and try to preserve more fat instead of burning it off. So, the dieting process becomes counterproductive. But with a carb cycling program, the body rarely gets a chance to acclimate itself to the constantly changing numbers in carb consumption.

However, with that said, it's still important that you shift your cycle up every once in a while. Weight plateaus are very real, and they can still happen while you're on a carb cycling program. Keep in mind that it's a lot easier for a larger person than a smaller person to burn a certain number of calories. This is because a larger body requires more calories in order to sustain itself. So, over time, as you're losing more and more weight, your caloric needs change as well. With that, you have to adjust to your changing body too. When you notice that your carb cycling program isn't as effective as it used to be, it's time for you to shift the cycles and alter the numbers. This is the only way you're going to be able to break through the plateaus you will inevitably face.

Is Carb Cycling for You?

Now, you've already been exposed to the different principles behind carb cycling and the science behind it. However, it's normal if you're not entirely sold on carb cycling just yet. It would be irresponsible for you to just automatically buy into this concept without first taking the time to really understand the nuances involved in this diet program. This is especially true considering that there are loads of other diet programs out there that you can incorporate into your daily life. Perhaps, these diets might be better for you. That's not a problem. Again, it's all about finding something that works best for you.

Given that, there is still a lot for you to learn and discover about carb cycling in relation to whether or not it would be good for you. To help you make a decision on it, you might want to consider the pros and cons that are involved in carb cycling. Of course, when you put a particular dietary philosophy up against others, certain diets are going to have their own respective strengths and weaknesses. While carb cycling has indeed proven itself to be effective to a critical mass of people, there are still certain trade-offs when you compare it to other effective diet programs.

Pros of Carb Cycling

The first advantage of carb cycling is that it's very accessible and easy to grasp for a lot of people. Also, it's not as strict as most other mainstream diets, so it won't really intimidate a lot of people who aren't too fond of drastic lifestyle changes. Since there are still days that allot for high carb consumption, it won't really be too difficult for most people to get into.

The second pro of carb cycling is that it's very flexible. There isn't really a very strict and specific program that everyone has to follow. The key to making the carb cycling diet work for you is making sure that it is tailored to your lifestyle. So, if you have a very busy day due to your job, then that means that you don't really have the time to work out. On days like those, you can still be on a diet by designating it as a low-carb day.

Another big advantage of carb cycling is that it is able to provide the body with a metabolic system that is more optimized for weight loss and fat burn. To put it simply, losing weight is just a matter of cutting calories to make sure that you're using up more energy that you're eating. However, sustainable weight loss is a lot more complicated than that. Eventually, your body adapts to your eating habits. So, if you're minimizing your calories, your body is eventually going to catch on to what you're doing. As a result, it will slow down its metabolic rate, and that won't be good for your weight loss. However, through carb cycling, your body never gets a chance to acclimate itself to what you're doing. So, it never slows down its metabolic rate, and your weight loss is never compromised. You're not on continuous deprivation of carbohydrates when you do carb cycling. As a result, your body never really feels like it has to restrict metabolic output to maintain energy reserves.

One added pro of carb cycling is that it has proven to improve athletic performance. This might be a very appealing benefit to all the readers out there who are competitive athletes who really take their training and athletic performance seriously. One common struggle that most athletes face is trying to lose weight without compromising athletic performance. A lot of the time, when training sessions get more and more intense, athletes will have to nourish their bodies with copious amounts of food, especially carbohydrates. However, carbs are also known to lead to blood sugar spikes, and this can compromise one's weight loss goals. This is why carb cycling is so effective. It still supplies the athlete with a steady influx of carbohydrates as sustenance for their intense training. But the low-carb days act as counterweights to the high-carb days, so as to prevent weight gain and even stimulate weight loss.

Lastly, you won't really have to stop yourself from eating all of your favorite food. If you're craving a generous bowl of ice cream, then you can have some. Just make sure that you fit your ice cream into your high-carb day. Cutting out carbs in traditional diets can get really boring or limiting in the long run. Fortunately, with carb cycling, you are constantly mixing things up. So, you don't have too many restrictions that limit your options.

Cons of Carb Cycling

One of the biggest cons of carb cycling is actually a con for many other diets as well. It requires great discipline. You have to pay so much attention to planning your meals and making sure that your macro intake meets specific numbers. This might not necessarily be the best diet plan for people who are unwilling to put a lot of work and effort into the planning and preparation phase. The planning and preparation process for carb cycling diets can get really comprehensive. With most diets, people are generally eating the same amount of food every day of the week. But with carb cycling, the numbers can change from day to day. So, this means that meal plans under a carb cycling method will require another added layer of detail that you need to take into consideration. With traditional meal planning, something that you would have for lunch on Monday can also be something that you can have for lunch once or twice more throughout the week. However, with carb cycling, that might not be viable as the nutritional demands might be different.

Another con of carb cycling is the fatigue that comes with low-carb days. Certain people just aren't capable of functioning properly when they don't get their fill of carbs. This might be a problem for people who need to be on top of their game but need to stay strict with their low carb consumption on those days.

Lastly, you might not be getting some valuable nutrients that you would typically get from your carbs. Fruits are a big no-no during low-carb days. However, fruits are also great sources of vitamins and minerals that make you healthier. Given that, you might have to resort to more expensive low-carb nutritional supplements to make sure that you're still getting your fill of vitamins and minerals.

Should You Give It a Try?

To be completely blunt, carb cycling used to exclusively be used by serious athletes and bodybuilders. However, it has managed to amass a mainstream popularity and is being used even by people who only engage in exercise as a form of recreation. Again, there really is no *best* diet out there. There is only a diet that works best for you. So, is carb cycling the best one you can adopt for your own lifestyle? Well, in order to come to an answer to that question, there are a few things that you need to take into consideration.

First of all, you need to look at the overall state of your health. Carb cycling might not necessarily be the healthiest option for people who are dealing with specific physical conditions. For instance, people who have issues with their blood sugar, such as diabetes or hypoglycemia, should definitely consult with their physician before taking on a diet like this. Remember that engaging in a dramatic carb-cutting diet can really alter the blood sugar spikes of your body, and this might be dangerous to you if you have a blood-related physical condition.

In addition to that, it might not be a good idea for you to

engage in this diet program if you're currently engaged in another dietary program. For example, you might be doing intermittent fasting and you're finding success in it. So, you don't want to give up intermittent fasting, but you also want to try carb cycling. Combining dietary philosophies like these might not necessarily be the healthiest thing for you or your body.

Final Thoughts

So, that's just a general overview of what carb cycling is. Of course, this was just a very brief run through of carb cycling. If you're really looking to try it out for yourself, you need to read more about it in this book. Ideally, by now, you will have come to a more educated opinion on whether this would be a great diet for you to try out. However, the best advice that you can get on this would be to just try it out. You really have nothing to lose so long as you know that your body will be able to handle it in a healthy manner. If it turns out that you don't like the diet or it doesn't really work for you, then you can always just abandon it and try something else. However, there is a lot of upside if you find out that it really does work for you and is effective. At the end of the day, embracing fitness and health is a journey. It's an exploration. It's continuous learning and self-discovery. And as the cliché goes, if you never try, then you'll never know.

Chapter 2:
Tailoring It to Women

Again, this isn't going to be just another cookie-cutter diet book that's going to assume that all of its readers are the same and are going to reap similar results. With dieting, it's very complex. What works for one isn't necessarily going to work the same way for another. In this sense, it's very important to streamline audiences. It's important to taper the prescription according to the needs of a patient. And in this case, the audience is women.

First of all, it's important to stress that this book is not being written because women are unfit to do the same things that men are capable of doing. That's not the message that is being sent out here. Of course, women always have the capacity to match and even surpass men in terms of ability and achievement. However, it would be foolish to assume that there are no biological differences between men and women. At its core, the whole idea of genders is founded on the fact that men and women have different physical makeups. To put it simply, men and women are wired differently when it comes to their physiques. So, as a result, men and women don't necessarily undergo the same bodily processes. This means that dietary programs like carb cycling aren't going to show pure consistency from person to person.

What this chapter is going to try to do is to shed more light on why carb cycling is different for women and why the approach has to be different as well. Again, when it comes to health and wellness, there are a lot of little details that need to be tended to. You might think that carb cycling would be a principle that would provide consistent results regardless of gender. But that isn't the case. Again, there are just too many variables that impact the effectiveness of a diet. One of those variables is gender. This is especially true if your ultimate goal is weight loss. Keep in mind that hormones play a very big role when it comes to metabolism and weight loss. It's also known that women undergo more hormonal changes and fluctuations than men do. That's just one aspect of why gender plays a big role in determining the effectiveness of the diet.

Ultimately, the goal of this chapter isn't to create division or any kind of discrimination. Rather, it's to take a more nuanced approach to talking about this diet. Again, when it comes to dietary programs like these, the devil is in the details. In order for you to properly execute this diet, then you need a more comprehensive overview of the gender-centric nuances that exist.

Why Carb Cycling Is Different for Women

We've already established how carb cycling is essentially just the science of inducing weight loss through alternating high- and low-carb days. Through these alternating intervals, the human body is more optimized to metabolize food and induce proper caloric processing. When you are consistently exposing your system to low-carb days, your body has better insulin sensitivity. This will help you burn fat over a more sustainable period as your metabolic system becomes more streamlined.

However, it's very important to stress that carbs are not the enemy. In fact, there are so many women out there who need carbohydrates for their bodies to function properly. And it's absolutely essential that we stress that fact. Here are some benefits of carbohydrate consumption for women, to name a few:

- Carbs help regulate hormonal systems in women.
- Carbs aid in the recovery from hypothalamic amenorrhea.
- Carbs help alleviate complications from thyroid issues.
- Carbs are essential for healthy pregnancies, etc.

So, while carbs may contribute to weight gain to a certain degree, just eliminating them altogether wouldn't necessarily be the smartest thing to do in most cases. Given that, carb cycling offers a perceivably safe middle ground. You're not eliminating carbs from your diet, but you're meticulously controlling your consumption so as to not interfere with your desires to lose weight.

However, there is a very common mistake that most women make when they try to get into carb cycling. They don't take their gender into consideration when doing so. This is understandable. When you take a look at the fitness industry, it has a tendency to be a very male-dominated community, especially when it comes to carb cycling. This is because, as we mentioned, carb cycling originated as a dieting technique for bodybuilders and high-profile athletes. As you may already know, those fields tend to have larger male communities. So, as this diet emerged into the mainstream, more women started adopting the carb cycling diet for themselves not knowing that they needed to factor their gender into the equation.

If you are a woman who is just trying to get into carb cycling for the first time and you don't really have a female resource person to help you out with things, don't fret. This segment of the book is going to equip you with some basic information that you just need to implant at the back of your mind as you make your way through this carb cycling journey.

The Protection of the Thyroid

We already touched on how the thyroid hormone is a very important component for fat loss. A high level of thyroid hormones can help stimulate fat loss, but a low-carb diet can dramatically slow down the production of thyroid hormones. This detail is particularly important for women to keep in mind because they tend to have more sensitive thyroid behaviors and metabolism. During the low-carb days, it's important that women don't go overboard with their restrictions because it could negatively alter the production of thyroid hormones. Ideally, during low-carb days, women would still be consuming a little more than 50 grams of carbohydrates a day.

Female Insulin Sensitivity

When talking about the hormones that get affected by

carbohydrate consumption, one must never forget about estrogen and progesterone. You might not have thought about this before, but your menstrual cycle can also dramatically impact the way that your body metabolizes the food that you consume. Depending on where you are on your menstrual cycle, it's either the carbs that you eat get processed more efficiently or they might end up being reserved as fat storage. This is why it would be better for you to somehow merge your carb cycling schedule with your menstrual cycle.

Normally, a woman's estrogen levels would be at their highest during the first two weeks of a menstrual cycle. During these initial two weeks, progesterone levels would also be at their lowest. What this means for dieting is that the body is more efficient at processing carbohydrates during these periods. In the luteal phase of a menstrual cycle (the last two weeks after ovulation), progesterone levels rise to a higher degree. This means that the body isn't going to be able to process carbohydrates all that well. This is a natural phenomenon that might be familiar to diabetic women. Typically, women with diabetes have to increase their dosage of insulin during the luteal phase of their menstrual cycle due to their blood sugar levels being relatively higher than usual.

So, what does this all mean for when you decide to start carb cycling?

Given that your menstrual cycles dictate your body's insulin levels, it's important that you time your carb cycles appropriately. To find the most success with carb cycling, it is advised that you reduce the amount of carbohydrates that you eat during the luteal phase or the last two weeks of your menstrual cycle. This is the period wherein your insulin sensitivity is going to be at its lowest, and it's important that you adjust your carb intake levels accordingly. So, given that you have to be very strict with your carb intake during your luteal phase, you have more liberty and freedom during the first two weeks of your cycle.

Of course, for a beginner, this might seem a little too vague or ambiguous for you. So, if you're looking for a real number that you can choose to work with, it would be best if you shoot for around 150 to 200 grams of carbohydrates every day for the first two weeks of your carb cycling. During the second week of the cycle, you even have the freedom to bump it up to around 220 to 250 grams of carbohydrates depending on your physical activity.

For the final two weeks of the cycle, this is where you have to start to taper your carb consumption significantly. You might want to consider dropping your carb intake to around a little over half of the amount that you were consuming during the initial two weeks. However, it's important that you don't overdo it by consistently going below 100 grams of carbs per day. This might impact your ability to conceive and also aggravate your thyroid issues.

Getting Fit for Women

As far as exercising is concerned, it shouldn't be something that you are wary of or be intimidated by. In fact, no matter what your gender, you should always make it a point to incorporate a healthy exercise routine into your daily life. Regular exercise is not only safe for everyone, but it's something that should be encouraged among all people. It's merely a matter of adopting an exercise routine or regimen that is well-suited for your lifestyle and biomechanical makeup. If you're doing carb cycling, then it's advisable for you to definitely incorporate exercise into your routine to maximize the effects of your diet.

Given that we've already talked about how your menstrual cycle can impact the effectiveness of your dieting, it shouldn't come as a surprise to you that it can affect the effectiveness of your training as well. To get straight to the point, during the initial two weeks of your cycle, you should engage in training that is more aerobic in nature. This means that your workouts should be performed at medium intensity, and they should be sustained for a relatively long period of time. Again, during your first two weeks, your carb intake is at your highest. This is why it's a good idea for you to push yourself with the length and duration of your workouts. It's not so much about increasing intensity. It's just about managing your energy well so that you are expending copious amounts of it over a sustained period. Don't be afraid to really push yourself as this is the phase of your cycle wherein your body is really primed to handle stressful physical conditions.

For the final two weeks of your cycle, this is where you want to consider just engaging in exercises that are more anaerobic in nature. Again, your carb intake is very low, and you might not have enough energy to sustain long and grueling training sessions. However, in order to compensate for the drop in workout durations, you have to make up for it with intensity. You should aim to get to around 80% to 90% of your maximum heart rate during these training periods. They don't have to last as long, but your training sessions have to leave you feeling like you gave it everything you've got in a short span of time. Some examples of anaerobic exercises are weightlifting, high intensity interval training, sprint intervals, and the like. Another added benefit of engaging in intense exercise sessions is that it helps sharpen your insulin sensitivity during this phase of your cycle. This means that you are able to burn and process fat more efficiently throughout the day even when you're no longer working out.

Mastering the Art of Cycle Syncing

All right, so a lot of important concepts have been laid out so far, and hopefully, they were able to provide you some deep insight into how your menstrual cycle affects your body. However, it can be very easy to just be overwhelmed by all of that info to the point that you end up forgetting some vital aspects of it. But in reality, it's all very simple. If you really want a more general overview of the important concepts behind syncing your carb and menstrual cycles, just remember that your typical menstrual cycle in relation to your carb cycle is made up of four different phases: menstrual, follicular, ovulatory, and luteal. The way that you eat and the way that you exercise should be dependent on which phase of the cycle you are currently in.

There are definitely some key concepts that you need to pay attention to with regards to syncing your dietary cycles and your menstrual cycles. And in order for you to really get the most out of your diet, you have to be willing to go the extra mile by paying close attention to all of the details. In order to systemize the planning process for you, it might be a good idea to take a phase-by-phase approach to discussing the ins and outs of cycle syncing.

Benefits of Cycle Syncing

If you're still in need of further convincing on why cycle syncing is going to serve you and your body well, then here are a few things that might incentivize you to really take this concept seriously. Aside from promoting weight loss and optimal athletic performance, carb cycling can also:

- minimize the effects of PMS or menstrual cramps
- decrease the chances of you getting hormonal acne
- balance your hormones after using a pill or IUD

- regulate your period if you have amenorrhea

- regulate your postpartum hormones

- minimize or eliminate the symptoms of PCOS

- optimize your body for conception

Foods to Avoid for Cycle Syncing

We've already discussed how there are certain foods that you should always try to have during certain phases of your cycle. However, before we get into the specifics of the food that you HAVE to eat, it's important to discuss the food that you have to eliminate altogether. Unfortunately, there are just certain popular food items out there that are loved by many but can wreak absolute chaos on hormone levels. Of course, depending on your age and fitness level, you might be able to get away with sneaking a few servings of these *banned* treats every once in a while. But for the most part, if you really want to make the most out of your diet, stay as strict as possible by avoiding these foods:

- processed and refined foods with non-natural ingredients

- white sugar

- margarine

- processed meats such as cold cuts and hot dogs

- canned goods

- deep-fried fast food

- hydrogenated oils

- soda

- high fructose corn syrup and other artificial sweeteners

Finding Your Phase

When it comes to cycle syncing, timing is everything. All of it hinges on you knowing which phase of your menstrual cycle you are in. If you are someone who has a regular cycle, then you stand to benefit from using an app that can help you track where you are. However, the general rule of thumb is that the first day of your menstrual cycle is also the day of your first big flow of blood. Things can get a little tricky when you have an irregular cycle. If you have an irregular cycle, it doesn't mean that you won't be able to reap the benefits of cycle syncing. Instead of relying on your menstrual cycle, you can use the lunar phases as a reference. If you haven't noticed, the lunar cycle also lasts for 28 days, much like a menstrual cycle. You can make use of various apps or internet sources to help you keep track of the lunar phases.

Menstrual Phase

The main thing that takes place on the first day of your menstrual phase is the shedding of the lining of your uterus. This takes place after your hormone levels drop, and this sends a signal to the tissues that are lining your uterus to shed and exit the body. In most cases, before the 7th day of the menstrual phase, the bleeding will have ceased. In the lead-up to this time, follicles are developed on the ovaries, and these contain eggs that are waiting to be fertilized.

But why does any of that information matter when it comes to plotting your diet?

This is because all of the hormonal changes taking place in your body during the menstrual phase are going to impact your energy levels dramatically. This is because your body will be depleted of estrogen at the start of the phase and will gradually rise up towards the end of it. You are also going to experience some iron deficiency as a result of all the blood that you're losing. Given that, you want to make sure that your diet is one that is rich in iron. Also, try consuming foods that help reduce inflammation to minimize the discomforts of menstruation.

So, when you're planning your diet for the menstrual phase, make sure to incorporate a lot of food that is warm and comforting. Go for a lot of soups, broths, casseroles, or stews that don't have too many harsh ingredients but are still filling and nutritious.

Follicular Phase

The follicular phase of the menstrual cycle typically lasts from days 7 to 14. It's during this phase wherein the estrogen and testosterone levels in the body will rise continuously while the linings of the uterus wall will start to thicken again. During the follicular phase, expect to feel somewhat energized, especially compared to how you were feeling in the menstrual phase. In this phase, you should take most of the energy that you're feeling to really go hard at the gym or wherever your workouts are. Really try to push yourself as this is usually the time of the month when you will be your strongest.

Typically, this is also going to be the phase where your body will be primed to burn up large amounts of calories. Don't be afraid to indulge in a lot of healthy carbohydrates, but also make sure that you are capitalizing on protein and fat intake as well. If you are a bodybuilder, then this is the time of the month for you to move some serious weight. And if you're putting the work in the gym, then make sure that you reward yourself with food. To be more specific, go for a lot of lean meats, healthy oils, fruits, and vegetables.

Ovulation Phase

After the follicular phase, the egg will travel down the fallopian tubes, making its way to the uterus. If the egg happens to meet sperm there, then the egg will become fertilized and travel down the tube even further to attach itself to the lining of the uterus. Coming from the highs of the follicular phase, you will experience a lot of grogginess and sluggishness here in the ovulation phase. You might also experience some bloating and it's possible that you will gain some weight during this period. However, you shouldn't worry much. It's probably just water weight as the result of the rising progesterone levels in your body.

Generally, you are going to want to focus on consuming a lot of fiber during this phase to ease any discomfort in your digestive system. Go for fruits and vegetables that are rich in fiber to aid your bowel movement. Also, it's very likely that your sugar level will drop during this phase. So, you want to make sure that you're still filling yourself up with a healthy dose of carbohydrates to balance your insulin levels out and keep yourself energized. However, avoid any carbohydrates that are too complex or strenuous to process such as wheats, grains, or pastas. For your training, stick to aerobic exercises that are performed at medium intensity. It's likely that you are going to burn way more calories during this phase with aerobic exercises.

Luteal Phase

The luteal phase is also the final phase of the menstrual cycle before the blood starts flowing again. During this phase, the uterus lining will really thicken itself up before it starts shedding itself in the menstrual phase. If the egg has not been fertilized by sperm, the estrogen and progesterone levels of the body will decrease, and this will signal the start of a new menstrual cycle. The egg will break away from the lining of the uterus, and it will also be shed during the next period.

Expect to feel really tired and moody during this phase. Your body is using up a lot of energy to gear up for a new menstrual cycle. As a result, there isn't really all that much energy left for you to do other things. Also, your serotonin levels will drop together with your estrogen. Remember that serotonin is a mood-balancing hormone. When your serotonin is compromised, it can be easy for you to feel overwhelmed by all of your feelings and emotions. Fortunately, exercise can help trigger the release of endorphins in your body, and this can help offset the dwindling levels of serotonin. After all, endorphins are known to be the natural happy hormones.

Also, since you don't have much energy to sustain long and grueling workouts, opt for shorter but more intense ones instead. This way, you are still getting the benefits of a full workout without having to use up too much of your stamina for it.

Final Thoughts

So as long as you remember those key points about the different phases of your menstrual cycle, you should do fine. Yes, it can be very complicated at the start to develop a plan that's going to work well for you. However, with more experience and experimentation, you will be able to drill your routine down to a tee. It's just a matter of staying patient and resilient with the diet. You shouldn't expect to get everything right on the first try. Make sure that you don't grow frustrated at the first signs of adversity. It's important that you stick with it and trust the process. Eventually, the results are going to come. You just can't rush and bypass the important aspects of the initial phases of carb cycling.

You might think that being a woman puts you at a disadvantage with your carb cycling because there are so many additional things that you need to keep track of. However, that isn't necessarily the case. In fact, you can use all of this extra knowledge and information to your advantage to really maximize the benefits of employing a carb cycling scheme for yourself.

Chapter 3:
Principles Behind Planning

We are very close to you getting to plot your own carb cycling plan. You have already been exposed to the many ways in which carb cycling is going to be different for you as compared to men. Of course, this new information might have complicated things a bit. But, at the very least, you are now armed with some of the knowledge that is necessary to make a more holistic and well-rounded plan for yourself. Again, remember that being a woman doesn't necessarily mean that you are at a disadvantage when it comes to your weight loss goals. It merely means that there are different things that you need to be keeping track of as far as variables and factors are concerned.

Now, it's time to tackle some concepts and principles that can be considered as commonalities between men and women. Again, we are very close to having you create your own plan. But before we get there, you have to familiarize yourself with a few important concepts and principles about the planning method. Remember, it's not just about randomly picking days where you consume large amounts of carbs or low amounts of carbs. It's also not just about randomly deciding on which number constitutes high and low consumption sizes either. There is a real mathematical science to it with rules that you need to adhere to if you want the diet to be effective.

Consider this chapter to be the final phase of the theoretical portion of this book. Soon, you are going to get a lot of practical tips and even a real opportunity to create your own plan for yourself. But first, it's very important that you really drill these important concepts and principles into your mind first. In this chapter, you will be given a very detailed breakdown of the principles of macro-counting and why it's important for you to do the math when determining your meal plan. Also, you will be briefed on some very basic principles that concern your developing a real diet plan for yourself. And at the end of this chapter, you will be given a sample meal plan that you can use to model your own diet plan after.

By the end of this chapter, you should be armed with all of the theoretical knowledge that you need to develop an effective carb cycling plan for yourself. You might be getting really fed up with a lot of these concepts, and that's understandable. However, you must also accept that losing serious weight over a sustainable period isn't just a matter of you winging it and hoping for the best. The reason that a lot of people struggle with losing weight is because it's a difficult endeavor, and it requires a lot of attention to detail. You need to have the patience that is necessary for you to gather all of the information that you need in order for you to be as educated as possible prior to putting things into practice.

Breaking the Cycle Down According to Macros

This may not necessarily be the first time that you've encountered the idea of counting *macros* for dieting. In fact, there is a very popular diet plan called IIFYM, or *If It Fits Your Macros,* and a lot of people actually swear by this dieting philosophy. This method of dieting is also known as flexible dieting as it doesn't really disallow people from certain foods. Rather, it limits one from overindulging in particular food types. This might all seem really vague right now, but you'll understand it more along the way.

What Are Macros?

First, we need to talk more in-depth about what macros are before we start talking about how you can count them and why they factor into your carb cycles. Macros or *macronutrients* are the three major nutrients that make up the bulk of the food that you eat on a daily basis to nourish yourself. The three macronutrients are protein, carbs, and fat. Each macro is going to have a corresponding caloric value, and they all serve different purposes in nourishing the human body. There are some foods that will have generous doses of each macronutrient. However, most of the time, a food item will only be biased towards just one or two macros. For example, most meats are heavy in protein and fat. Wheats and grains are mostly loaded with carbohydrates. Oils are almost exclusively made up of fat. In order for your body to function optimally, you need appropriate doses of each macronutrient. So, let's break down the three macros, shall we?

Carbohydrates. No, they're not the enemy. Forget everything that you've been told about carbs. A lot of the time, when the mainstream media tries to come up with marketing campaigns to scare people into getting fit, they depict images of overweight people munching down on carb-rich food like ice cream, doughnuts, pizza, and whatnot. Sure, it's true that an overindulgence in carbohydrates can make a person fat. But you can also say the same for any other macronutrient as well. There really isn't much sense in singling out carbohydrates as a macronutrient that needs to be avoided at all costs. Remember, weight loss or weight gain is all a matter of calories going in or out of the body. And a single gram of carbohydrates is going to carry around 4 calories. One gram of carbohydrates carries the same caloric value as a single gram of protein. And yet, carbohydrates are hailed as the devil, and protein is propped up to be *the* health macro. Keep in mind that carbs are responsible for fueling the body with energy. You wouldn't be able to work out at the gym or train on the track at an optimal level if you didn't have any carbs in your system. When you eat carbs, your body processes them into glucose, which serves as the source of your body's energy to do everything that it needs to function properly. However, when there is excess energy leftover, it then gets converted as stored fat. This is the reason why overconsumption of carbs is bad and why this macro often gets a bad rap in the fitness community.

Fats. Next up, there are fats. Fat is actually another macronutrient that is known to have a bad rap in the fitness community. When carb-heavy foods like doughnuts or chocolates aren't being demonized in mainstream media, it's usually fat-heavy food like fried chicken, cheeseburgers, and fast food items. However, unlike carbohydrates, there is some validity to the demonization of fats due to its caloric values. A single gram of fat carries a whopping 9 calories. But that doesn't mean that fat is a macro that should be avoided at all costs. Again, it's just a matter of managing the consumption of fat so as to not fall into the trap of overindulgence. Fats are vital to the normal and healthy function of a human body.

Contrary to what most people are led to believe, eating fat won't necessarily translate to you also getting fat. This myth has already been debunked by the success of the keto diet, a fat-centric diet that stimulates weight loss. However, there are just certain fat-heavy foods that have little nutritional value and might lead to the surplus of calories which can eventually lead to weight gain. Examples of unhealthy fat sources are vegetable oils, margarine, and fast food, which are very bad for the body. But on the other side of the spectrum, there are healthy fat sources like avocados, coconut oil, nuts, nut butters, and more that offer a lot of nutritional value. Fats like these are responsible for making sure that the body is able to efficiently absorb and process nutrients in the body. On top of that, fats aid in hormone and body temperature regulation as well.

Protein. Lastly, there is protein. This is the macronutrient that is most often heralded as the ideal poster child for health and wellness. And it's really not all that hard to see why. Regardless of whatever your fitness goals might be, it's always important that you incorporate a generous allocation of protein into your diet. As with carbohydrates, proteins only have 4 calories for every gram. This means that you have more liberty to eat more of it without having to worry about going into a caloric surplus. Also, this is the macronutrient that is responsible for building the muscular cells and tissues in your body. This is precisely the reason why protein is the go-to macro for serious athletes like weightlifters, bodybuilders, runners, and more. Protein is a macronutrient that is most commonly found in meat, beans, seafood, and poultry to name a few.

Determining Your TDEE or Total Daily Energy Expenditure

Now, just because you know what macros are doesn't mean

that you can get started on determining how much of them you need to eat. There is one last step that you need to perform before you can calculate your recommended macro numbers. You must first find out what your *TDEE* or total daily energy expenditure is. Don't worry. It isn't going to require you to do a lot of heavy math. In fact, it's merely a matter of inputting some values into a calculator that you can find online and have the computer do the work for you. The calculator found at https://tdeecalculator.net/ is a perfect one that you can use. Essentially, the TDEE is a determination of how many calories you are using up every day based on your age, body composition, and level of your physical activity.

Your body typically has a base metabolic rate or a BMR. This is essentially how many calories your body will burn while it's at rest. Your BMR is computed based on your physical composition and your age. However, the TDEE is a more comprehensive evaluation of how many calories you are burning every day as it takes into consideration your level of physical activity as well. The reason why it's important for you to learn your TDEE is because it gives you a solid number to work with when figuring out the distribution of your macros.

So, whatever result you get for your TDEE calculation is essentially the number of calories that you need to eat every day to maintain your weight. In order for you to lose or gain weight, you need to get in either a caloric deficit or surplus, respectively. One pound of fat approximates to around 3,500 calories. So, if you want to lose one pound of fat, you are going to have to get into a caloric deficit of 3,500 calories. Obviously, it wouldn't be practical for regular folk to be getting into a deficit of 3,500 calories every single day. This is only a number that is achievable for the highest-level athletes who train multiple hours in a day. For the most part, people should only shoot for a caloric deficit of around 500 to 1,000 calories per day. This should enable you to lose 1 to 2 pounds a week. So, let's say that based on your TDEE calculation, you are burning 2,200 calories every day. If you restrict yourself to eating just 1,200 calories per day, you will eventually lose 2 pounds within a span of a week. However, take note that this is not an exact science and that there is a chance that you will lose more or less weight than is expected. There really is no way that you can accurately gauge just how many calories you burn on any given day. But the TDEE calculator should give you a fairly good idea of a ballpark number that you can use as a guide. Also, make sure your target daily caloric deficit doesn't fall outside the 500 to 1,000 calorie range. Sure, you can try to exceed that if you're looking to lose a huge amount of weight quickly. However, that wouldn't be a healthy or a sustainable way to go about weight loss.

Calculating Your Macros

Again, calories don't necessarily tell the whole story. Sure, in essence, you would be able to lose weight by merely tracking your calories alone. But a more holistic approach to health and wellness requires you to actively and accurately track your macros. However, tracking your macros requires you to know your TDCI or target daily caloric intake. You will learn more about how to compute your ideal TDCI later on in the book., You need to use your TDCI as a foundation to build your macro consumption breakdown. If we go back to the example that was used in the previous step, you might limit yourself to just 1,200 calories per day so that you can lose 2 pounds a week. So, based on that, your TDCI would be 1,200 calories. The breakdown of your macros should be based on this number.

Ideally, this is how you want to distribute your macros:

Your carbs should make up around 40-60% of your calories.

Fats should make up 20-30% of calories. And protein should make up 20-40% of calories. Earlier, we learned that every gram of each macro is going to carry a corresponding caloric value. Carbs and proteins have 4 calories each for every gram, and fats have 9 calories for every gram. To determine how many grams of each macro you need to eat, you just have to divide the caloric allocation you have for each macro by its corresponding caloric value. Don't worry, all of this might be a little difficult to imagine for now, so let's try to put these formulas to work.

Let's say, that based on the recommended caloric allocations, you have decided to break down your macros into 50% carbs, 30% protein, and 20% fat. So, based on those values together with your TDCI, this is how the distribution of your macros should look:

Total Carbs = 1,200 * 0.5 = 600 / 4 = 150 grams

Total Protein = 1,200 * 0.3 = 360 / 4 = 90 grams

Total Fat = 1,200 * 0.2 = 240 / 9 = 26.7 grams

Of course, this is just a general recommendation and example of what someone's daily macro distribution and consumption could look like. However, as mentioned, this book isn't about to give you a cookie-cutter recommendation. If you are reading this book, you are a woman who wants to lose weight through carb cycling. With that, there are specific numbers that you should be hitting in order for you to achieve your goals. And as mentioned, when you are carb cycling, you aren't eating the same amount of carbs every day.

Ideal Macros for High and Low Days

So, now you have the formula for computing your macros. It wasn't all that hard, right? If the manual computations really trouble you, feel free to make use of various tools or apps that you can find on your phone or on the internet to help you out. In any case, knowing how to compute your ideal macros is only part of the battle. Now, you have to figure out how to adjust your macro distribution based on your high- and low-carb days.

Just for a quick refresher, when you are carb cycling, you are essentially giving yourself intervals for your carb consumption. There are certain days in which you should be taking relatively high amounts of carbohydrates, and there should be days where you are taking low amounts. Determining which days of the week should be your high or low ones is a topic that will be discussed in the latter parts of this chapter. For now, you have to figure out how you're going to compute your macros relative to your high and low days. The example that was given previously was merely a format for someone who was tracking macros without going through carb cycling. If we take that same example and apply carb cycling principles to it, this is how it would look:

For high-carb days, you want to make sure that this is where you really insert a bulk of your carb consumption throughout the week. However, all of the same principles of macro calculation apply. It's merely a matter of adjusting target values. In the previous example, only 50% of the TDCI was accounted for by carbohydrates. Maybe, on high-carb days, you can bump that number up to 55% or even 60%. Your decision will depend on your level of physical activity or on whatever works for you. So, since you bumped your carb allocation up to 55%, doesn't that mean that you would be exceeding your TDCI? Yes, that is true. This is why one or both of the other macros should adjust. Of course, you can adjust the numbers based on your own personal preference. However, if you're a beginner and you don't know how to go about those adjustments, the general rule of thumb is that when your carbs go up, your fat should go down, and vice-versa. The protein consumption should remain relatively consistent on both high- and low-carb days. So, on high-carb days, if you're increasing consumption of carbs by around 5%, then that means you need to take 5% of calories away from your fat consumption. Based on the given example, the new macro distribution of your high-carb days should look like this:

Total Carbs = 1,200 * 0.55 = 660 / 4 = 165 grams

Total Protein = 1,200 * 0.3 = 360 / 4 = 90 grams

Total Fat = 1,200 * 0.15 = 180/ 9 = 20 grams

Again, this is just an example, and it's okay if your plan for high-carb days doesn't exactly look like this. This is merely an illustration of how you would adjust your macro distribution for high-carb days. Now, for your low-carb days, it's important that you really limit your carbs as much as possible. However, as has been previously mentioned, for women, it's important that you never consistently stray too far away from the 100 gram-threshold for minimum carb consumption. With the way that your body is wired, it's important that you don't deprive yourself of carbs too much in order for your body to function properly. So, if on high-carb days, you are looking to increase your average carb consumption by 5%, maybe it would be okay for you to decrease your carbs by 10% on low-carb days. Let's see what that looks like:

Total Carbs = 1,200 * 0.40 = 480/ 4 = 120 grams

Total Protein = 1,200 * 0.3 = 360 / 4 = 90 grams

Total Fat = 1,200 * 0.3 = 360 / 9 = 40 grams

With this example, you are staying within the safe zone for minimal carb consumption as a woman. However, feel free to push the envelope even further if you're up for the challenge.

Try to gradually lower your carb consumption on low-carb days and see how it works for you. If your body responds well and you're feeling fine, then keep it up. If you start feeling sluggish and too tired over an extended period of time, it might be a sign that you're not eating enough. So, again, it's important for you to really listen to your body.

Let's try to change the values a little bit as we illustrate another example. Imagine that you are a woman whose goal is to eat just 1,500 calories a day. For high-carb days, you have decided that you will be eating 60% carbs, 20% protein, and 20% fat. For low-carb days, you think that you would be able to handle 35% carbs, 30% protein, and 35% fat.

For high-carb days, this is how the computations should play out:

Total Carbs = 1,500 * 0.6 = 900 / 4 = 225 grams

Total Protein = 1,500 * 0.2 = 300 / 4 = 75 grams

Total Fat = 1,500 * 0.2 = 300 / 9 = 33.3 grams

For low-carb days, this is how much you would be eating:

Total Carbs = 1,500 * 0.35 = 525 / 4 = 131.25 grams

Total Protein = 1,500 * 0.3 = 500 / 4 = 125 grams

Total Fat = 1,500 * 0.35 = 525 / 9 = 58.3 grams

There you have it. Hopefully, you have a much clearer picture by now of how you would compute your macros for your high and low days. Yes, it might feel like a lot of work. However, most of this kind of work is only done at the start. Remember, you have been warned that carb cycling is going to have a very meticulous planning process. But at the very least, if you develop a plan that works and you manage to stick to it, you are undoubtedly going to yield favorable results.

How To Make a Diet Plan

Now, we've discussed all of the annoying numerical aspects of making your diet plan. You're probably all fed up with all of these numbers and computations by now. Don't worry. That aspect of the planning and preparation process is over. Now, it's time to really develop your plan and figure out how to plot your low- and high-carb days. Of course, given that you are the architect of your own plan, this is where you have more freedom to really experiment and play around with what is going to work best for you. There are many different possible approaches that you could take to making your carb cycling plan. Some people choose to alternate on a daily basis. There are those who go a few days on high and a few days on low. There are also those who take a weekly interval approach to cycling. Again, it really depends on what kind of person you are and the lifestyle that you have.

However, for you, the reader, a woman who is looking to lose weight, we need to take a more specialized approach to determining your carb cycle. In a previous chapter, we talked about how it would be ideal for you to synchronize your carb and menstrual cycles in order to make the most out of your diet. So, we will integrate those principles into making your plan. Also, make sure that you incorporate some level of exercise into your plan as well. Hopefully, if you are reading, you are still physically able to move athletically to the point that you are capable of exercising or working out. It doesn't matter if you have a very low level of fitness. So as long as you have the capacity to move, you should be exercising. Heck, even a quick internet search will show you videos of disabled or differently-abled people doing some of the most intense workouts you will ever see. There's no excuse there. If you are serious about losing weight, then you need to exercise.

This is going to be a sample diet and exercise plan that you can use if you are looking to synchronize your menstrual cycle together with your diet and fitness regimen. Again, remember that you are going to want to shoot for high-carb days during the first two weeks of the cycle and then taper off towards the final two weeks. If you need a refresher on this, feel free to return back to the second chapter discussing how your menstrual cycle impacts your insulin sensitivity levels. In any case, here is a recommended carb cycling diet plan that takes into consideration your level of exercise output and menstrual cycle for a woman who is eating 1,500 calories per day.

Day 1: low carbs (125 grams) with high volume training

Day 2: high carbs (230 grams) with high volume training

Day 3: high carbs (200 grams) with high volume training

Day 4: low carbs (115 grams) with minimal training/active recovery

Day 5: high carbs (220 grams) with high volume training

Day 6: high carbs (220 grams) with high intensity training

Day 7: low carbs (100 grams) with minimal training/active recovery

Day 8: medium-high (180 grams) carbs with high intensity training

Day 9: high carbs (200 grams) with high volume training

Day 10: high carbs (215 grams) with high volume training

Day 11: high carbs (220 grams) with high volume training

Day 12: high carbs (200 grams) with high intensity training

Day 13: low carbs (115 grams) with minimal training/active recovery

Day 14: high carbs (195 grams) with high volume training

Day 15: medium-high (180 grams) carbs with high intensity training

Day 16: low carbs (125 grams) with high intensity training

Day 17: low carbs (100 grams) with high intensity training

Day 18: low carbs (130 grams) with minimal training/active recovery

Day 19: low carbs (120 grams) with high intensity training

Day 20: low carbs (125 grams) with moderate intensity training

Day 21: low carbs (125 grams) with minimal training/active recovery

Day 22: low carbs (140 grams) with moderate intensity training

Day 23: low carbs (120 grams) with moderate intensity training

Day 24: low carbs (125 grams) with minimal training/active recovery

Day 25: medium carbs (185 grams) with high intensity training

Day 26: low carbs (130 grams) with high intensity training

Day 27: low carbs (125 grams) with high intensity training

Day 28: low carbs (120 grams) with minimal training/active recovery

Again, this is merely a sample plan that you can choose to adopt for yourself. Of course, since this is your diet plan, only you can determine if it works for you or not. Don't be afraid to fine-tune this plan as you go to better suit your lifestyle. Remember that a lot of what makes a diet sustainable is dependent on whether the dieter enjoys executing it or not.

This book might serve as an authority figure or valuable resource in helping you shape your path, but it's still ultimately your own path. There is no *one way* to achieve weight loss for women through carb cycling. There is plenty of room for experimentation and trial-and-error here. Feel free to tweak this recommended plan however you see fit.

Sample Weekly Meal Plan

Of course, it's not enough that this book advises you on which days you should be having high carbs and low carbs. You need to gain better insight into what the meals for those days should look like as well. For this part of the chapter, we are going to look into some concrete meal plans that you can use for your high- and low-carb distributions. For the purposes of this sample meal plan, we will assume the following format for carb cycling over a seven-day cycle:

Low-High-High-Low-High-High-Low

Day 1: Low-Carb Day

Breakfast: 4-Egg and Cheese Omelette with Toast Slices

Calories: 383 kcal, Carbs: 36 g, Fat: 17 g, Protein: 21 g

Lunch: Zucchini and Walnut Salad

Calories: 595 kcal, Carbs: 8 g, Fat: 58 g, Protein: 9 g

Snacks: Almond Milkshake

Calories: 264 kcal, Carbs: 20 g, Fat: 16 g, Protein: 14 g

Dinner: Turkey Sandwich on Whole Wheat

Calories: 241 kcal, Carbs: 36 g, Fat: 4.5 g, Protein: 15.5 g

Day 2: High-Carb Day

Breakfast: Baked Mushroom and Egg with Chicken and Multigrain Rice

Calories: 600 kcal, Carbs: 47 g, Fat: 24 g, Protein: 47 g

Lunch: Peanut Orange Chicken with Vegetables and Rice

Calories: 602 kcal, Carbs: 47 g, Fat: 24 g, Protein: 50 g

Snacks: Peanut Butter Sandwich on Wheat Bread

Calories: 327 kcal, Carbs: 30 g, Fat: 18 g, Protein: 15 g

Dinner: Sweet and Spicy Beef Bowl

Calories: 459 kcal, Carbs: 45 g, Fat: 11 g, Protein: 40 g

Day 3: High-Carb Day

Breakfast: Peanut Butter Banana Oatmeal with Egg and Pulled Pork

Calories: 603 kcal, Carbs: 47 g, Fat: g, Protein: 49 g

Lunch: Slow-Cooked Chicken and Rice Casserole

Calories: 380 kcal, Carbs: 36 g, Fat: 11 g, Protein: 36 g

Snacks: Multigrain Bread with Olive Oil

Calories: 257 kcal, Carbs: 22.6 g, Fat: 16.2 g, Protein: 7 g

Dinner: Turkey Sandwich on Whole Wheat

Calories: 241 kcal, Carbs: 36 g, Fat: 4.5 g, Protein: 15.5 g

Day 4: Low-Carb Day

Breakfast: Cream Cheese Pancakes

Calories: 344 kcal, Carbs: 3 g, Fat: 29 g, Protein: 17 g

Lunch: Turkey Sandwich on Whole Wheat

Calories: 241 kcal, Carbs: 36 g, Fat: 4.5 g, Protein: 15.5 g

Snacks: Low-Carb Deviled Eggs

Calories: 163 kcal, Carbs: 0.5 g, Fat: 15 g, Protein: 7 g

Dinner: Fried Kale and Broccoli Salad

Calories: 1,022 kcal, Carbs: 13 g, Fat: 94 g, Protein: 22 g

Day 5: High-Carb Day

Breakfast: Fruity Oatmeal Bowl (High Carb)

Calories: 348 kcal, Carbs: 59 g, Fat: 10 g, Protein:7 g

Lunch: Moroccan Couscous with Flank Steak

Calories: 371 kcal, Carbs: 41 g, Fat: 9 g, Protein: 32 g

Snacks: Multigrain Bread with Olive Oil

Calories: 257 kcal, Carbs: 22.6 g, Fat: 16.2 g, Protein: 7 g

Dinner: Slow-Cooked Chicken and Rice Casserole

Calories: 380 kcal, Carbs: 36 g, Fat: 11 g, Protein: 36 g

Day 6: High-Carb Day

Breakfast: Cream Cheese Pancakes

Calories: 344 kcal, Carbs: 3 g, Fat: 29 g, Protein: 17 g

Lunch: Spicy Avocado Chicken Salad Wrap

Calories: 534 kcal, Carbs: 49 g, Fat: 18 g, Protein: 47 g

Snacks: Peanut Butter Sandwich on Wheat Bread

Calories: 327 kcal, Carbs: 30 g, Fat: 18 g, Protein: 15

Dinner: Slow-Cooked Chicken and Rice Casserole

Calories: 380 kcal, Carbs: 36 g, Fat: 11 g, Protein: 36 g

Day 7: Low-Carb Day

Breakfast: Keto Coconut Porridge

Calories: 486 kcal, Carbs: 4 g, Fat: 49 g, Protein: 9 g

Lunch: Zucchini and Walnut Salad

Calories: 595 kcal, Carbs: 8 g, Fat: 58 g, Protein: 9 g

Snacks: 1 oz of Almonds

Calories: 163 kcal, Carbs: 12 g, Fat: 2 g, Protein: 11 g

Dinner: Salad in a Jar

Calories: 876 kcal, Carbs: 11 g, Fat: 76 g, Protein: 27 g

Final Thoughts

Again, these are just some very rough concepts that you can choose to adopt for your own personal diet plan. Regardless, all of the principles are laid out here, and they should serve as the foundation for your diet. At the end of the day, you are really going to have to get in there and make a few adjustments to better suit your own personal needs and goals. If you are looking to really follow this meal plan, you will find the recipes for these food items in another chapter towards the end of this book.

Author's Note

So, are you enjoying the book so far? Maybe you should take a quick breather and gather your thoughts for a bit. A lot of very deep and important concepts have already been covered, and you may need to take some time to reflect on them. Hopefully, you will have gained some profound insight into carb cycling by now. As an author, it would make me really happy to know that my words have added some degree of value to your life. In my line of work, reviews are really hard to come by, and they can really help push my career forward so that I can come up with more meaningful content like this to help you and other people as well.

With that, I wish you could just take the time right now to write a brief review of this book on Amazon. It doesn't have to be anything too complicated or anything. It just has to be honest. Any time that you spend to write a review would be greatly appreciated by me and many writers like myself. Thank you so much for reading this book and taking the time to write a review for it. It really means a lot to me. Now, onwards to the rest of the book!

Chapter 4:
Create Your Own Plan

Not to hype this chapter up, but everything that you have read so far in this book has led to this. It's now time for you to create your own diet plan for yourself. Consider this to be the output of everything that you've been working hard to learn up to this point. Yes, gaining knowledge and proficiency in theory is all well and good. It's important. However, none of that will be of value unless you are able to apply your lessons to your everyday life. And this chapter is going to guide you throughout that process.

It can't be emphasized enough that the planning and preparation phases of carb cycling might be the most important. It doesn't matter how strictly you execute your plan if it's a faulty one to begin with. When you seriously want to get into carb cycling, it's vital that you really take the time to sit down and develop a plan that is foolproof. So, before we get right into the thick of things with this chapter, a few reminders are warranted. Then, you should have some kind of documentation device ready as we proceed to the latter parts of this chapter where you will start developing your own plan.

It's not enough that this book just supplies you a comprehensively laid out plan that you can follow to the tee. Remember that this book's author has no knowledge of what kind of lifestyle you lead, how many hours you work, what level of fitness you have, and other such details. There are too many variables that need to be taken into consideration, and it's only you who has knowledge of those things. All that this book can provide you is a rough sketch or outline of the drawing that you need to finish. You just have to do the proper shading and coloring at this point.

Of course, you can always choose to go the easy route and merely adopt some kind of ready-made outline that is available online. A quick internet search will present you with a myriad of ready-made options that you can choose to follow on your own. You might be able to find success in it and you might not. Whatever the case, know that taking the time to really pay attention to all the details of fine-tuning your diet to your lifestyle will serve you better in the long run.

Think of your diet like it's a dress. When you go shopping for dresses, it's a lot of fun, right? You see different dresses that are fit for differently sized people, and they come in all sorts of shapes and colors. There are some dresses that you admire, but they don't fit you. And there are some dresses that might fit you really well, but you aren't really a fan of particular details like its colors or stitch patterns. But eventually, you are bound to find a dress that will be *okay* and do the job. You buy it and you look good in it. You make it work. But ultimately, you know that the dress isn't *perfect*.

That's the shopping equivalent of just taking a ready-made carb cycling pattern online and applying it to your own life. Sure, you can probably find something that you like and that will grant you some success. But buying a ready-to-wear dress is nothing compared to visiting a proper designer and creating a dress from scratch. By getting a dress designed specifically for you, you are granted the opportunity to pore over every single detail. You will have a say in the crafting of the dress from the start right to the finish. And the end product is bound to be something that you're happy with... all because you took the time to take a more active role in the planning and design process.

Think of this chapter as you are chatting with your designer about your dream dress. Except now, we're talking about your dream diet. Yes, there are certain rules and principles that you have to follow. And a lot of them have already been laid out here in this book. At this point, it's just a matter of taking everything that you learned and putting it all to paper (or jot it down on your phone if you're a techier person). Again, there is a lot of upside to decisively being the one who makes your diet plan from scratch. And if you're up for that challenge, this chapter is going to meticulously guide you through that process with a streamlined series of steps that you can follow to a tee.

But first... a few reminders.

Things to Remember When Making Your Own Diet Plan

Before we jump into the crafting of your specialized diet plan, there are a few things that you need to keep in mind first. Consider this segment of the chapter to be a short rehashing of everything that you have learned so far. It's important that you keep these guiding principles to heart so that you don't have to second-guess yourself throughout the entire process.

There Are Many Different Factors to Consider When Deciding on High and Low Intervals

When deciding on which days to designate as high-carb or low-carb days, there are a myriad of different factors that you need to consider. However, in order to simplify things for you, here are a few principles that you need to keep in mind:

- The heavier you are or bigger your current body mass, the more calories you are burning. So, you have a higher threshold for carb consumption than those who are smaller than you.

- On the days that you don't work out, you are burning fewer calories. So, it would be best if you designate these days as your low-carb days as well. This will help prevent weight gain even when you're not exercising.

- The more drastic your goals are, then the more drastic your carb cuts have to be. If you want to lose a large amount of weight in a short amount of time, then you need to seriously cut back on your calories. On high-carb days, make sure that you don't overindulge. On low-carb days, keep the numbers as low as you possibly can with your carb consumption.

- When your training for a particular day is aerobic in nature, feel free to have a high-carb day. Just make sure that your workouts are long enough for you to completely deplete your converted glucose. If your training day is more anaerobic or intense in nature, you will be able to get by with having a low-carb day.

- If you are training for a competition, be sure to factor your schedule into your diet plan. If you are training for a marathon, you will want to gradually increase your high-carb days as the competition nears. However, if you are training as a bodybuilder, you will want to have more low-carb days as you near the date of competition.

Carb Cycling Isn't the Same as Keto

While both dietary philosophies have you cutting down on carbs significantly to a certain degree, they don't necessarily trigger the same kind of processes in your body. With keto, you cut down on carbohydrates so that your body enters a ketogenic state. What this means is that your body has recognized a shortage of carbohydrates and has to search for alternative sources of energy. To do this, the body takes the fat reserves of the body and triggers the production of ketones in your liver. These ketones are then converted into the energy that is needed to fuel your body. By doing this, the body goes into an ultra-fat-burning mode in an effort to keep up with its own caloric demands.

On the other hand, with carb cycling, achieving ketosis isn't necessarily the end goal. Ultimately, the goal of carb cycling is to strengthen a body's insulin sensitivity while also achieving a caloric deficit in order to facilitate weight loss. Some of the side effects of carb cycling also include improved athletic performance and optimized digestive function.

Carb Cycling Is Different for Women than It Is for Men

This is the whole point of this book. Carb cycling is a process that can work for both men and women. However, there have to be different approaches for each gender. This is due to the fact that the hormonal makeup of men and women is fundamentally different. Keep in mind that the body's ability to burn fat is largely dependent on the state of one's hormone levels as well. When a carb cycling plan is not optimized for hormonal imbalances, then it might not be as effective as it should be.

It Would Be Best to Sync Carb and Menstrual Cycles

Studies have shown that a woman's hormone levels are heavily influenced by her menstrual cycle. So, in order to make the most out of a carb cycling dietary scheme, it is best to synchronize the carb cycle together with a woman's menstrual cycle. If you have irregular cycles, you can always opt to just synchronize your carb cycle with the lunar cycle instead.

On High-Carb Days, Eat Little Fat... and Vice-Versa

Ideally, you should aim for the same number of calories every day for you to lose weight. However, the makeup of your macro distribution should differ depending on whether you have a low-carb or a high-carb day. Regardless of whether you have a low-carb or high-carb day, your protein consumption should remain relatively consistent all throughout. The two macronutrients that you need to drastically adjust over the course of a cycle are your carbs and your fats. On high-carb days, make sure that you eat less fat. On low-carb days, eat more fat to make sure that you meet your daily caloric targets.

Don't Overcomplicate Things

Don't overcomplicate things. When you're developing your plan, there really is no need to make things more complicated than they already are. It's really just a matter of figuring out what days would better serve as low-carb or high-carb days. The math shouldn't be all that complicated either. All of the formulas have been laid out for you. You just have to input the values yourself and develop a plan around that. If all else fails, just remember KISS - keep it simple, sweetheart.

Step-by-Step Guide to Making Your Carb Cycling Plan

Do you have a pen and paper ready? It's time for you to start making your own carb cycling plan. Are you excited? You should be. This is a very important step that you are taking towards becoming the best and healthiest version of yourself. However, before you actually start putting your pen to paper, it's important to manage your expectations first. Be conscious of the fact that it's possible that the plan you come up with right now isn't necessarily going to give you the results that you want. Sometimes, you might not be losing as much weight as you want. In some instances, you might not even be losing weight at all. And in some rare cases, you might even find yourself gaining weight instead. If that's the case, don't give up. It's okay to be frustrated, but you shouldn't give up on the process entirely. Try to reassess your plan and make a few adjustments wherever you can. Ultimately, you shouldn't shy away from revisiting your plan in the future and tweaking things to make sure that your evolving needs are constantly being met.

With that said, let's proceed to the first step...

Step 1: Know Your Vital Statistics

First of all, you need to know your vital statistics. Obviously, this diet is a solution to a problem. You want to lose weight because you think that there is a problem with the current makeup of your body. However, it's not enough that you just think that you're overweight. You need to familiarize yourself with the numbers behind your body composition. At the very least, you should at least know how much you weigh before you start dieting. The number on the scale might not necessarily tell the whole story, but it definitely says a lot. Next, you must also know your BMI or body mass index.

There are those who will say that the BMI is an outdated measure of fitness and that it should be obsolete by now. And there is some truth to that. However, it can still serve as a somewhat accurate gauge of fitness for some people. If you really want to take things to another level, you can also get yourself measured for body fat percentage, VO2 max, and other health tests. The more you know about your body, then the better position you will be in to know what kind of work awaits you.

Step 2: Establish Your Goals

After step one, you should already have a good sense of where you are as far as your health and fitness levels are concerned. From this, you should be able to gather information on your potential points of improvement or problem area. For example, you might learn from your vital statistics that you are overweight and that you are at risk for heart disease, diabetes, or even cancer. So, you set a goal for yourself to lose a certain amount of weight just to make sure that you minimize your risk of contracting such complications. Perhaps you are already a relatively lean person, but you really want to try to chisel your body to allow your muscles to really shine. In order to do so, you have to lower your body fat percentage. Whatever the case, establishing a goal is very important. Your goal is going to serve as your *why* in everything that you do. This should be your primary mover and motivator to get the job done with your diet and training. Consider your goals to be your North Star. They are your guiding light. You can't just diet for the hell of it. In order to get anything substantial done in life, you must always be structured and purposeful with your actions.

Step 3: Set Your Training Regimen

This might be the step that a lot of you are going to show some level of hesitation with. This is especially true if you haven't really been athletic in your life. That's okay. It's normal to not be happy about the idea of having to develop a consistent training regimen. However, in order for you to really make the most out of your carb cycling diet, you have to be willing to exercise. The diet isn't going to work the way that it's supposed to if you don't take the time to incorporate exercise into your daily routine.

Of course, you don't have to train to be a superstar athlete or anything. You don't have to make it a point to spend hours on end at the gym. Experts say that the recommended time that you should be working out is at least 3 to 5 times a week for around 30 minutes to 1 hour per session. Ideally, you would elevate your heart rate to around 60% to 80% of your max heart rate during these sessions. This way, you are building cardiovascular strength, and you are also burning calories to facilitate weight loss at the same time.

Step 4: Find Your Total Daily Energy Expenditure (TDEE)

Another reason why you had to figure out your workout routine was so that you could have a more accurate gauge of your TDEE, or total daily energy expenditure. In order for you to figure out how much food you need to eat every day to lose weight, you have to figure out how many calories you are burning on a daily basis first. Now, keep in mind that different people burn different amounts of calories every day. There are plenty of factors that can help influence a body's metabolic output, such as body mass, level of physical activity, and age.

Also, there really is no accurate way for you to gauge how many calories you are burning. However, there is a calculator that you can make use of online to give you a rough estimate or a ballpark figure of how many calories you lose every day. This step has already been laid out in detail for you in a previous chapter of this book.

Step 5: Find Your Total Daily Caloric Intake

Once you've found out your TDEE, it's now time for you to compute your total daily caloric intake. This is where you begin to incorporate your goals, your vital stats, and your TDEE. All of the steps that preceded this one were vital for this particular computation. In this step, you have to figure out how much food you SHOULD be consuming every day in order for you to lose the amount of weight that you want. This is also called your total daily caloric intake or TDCI.

Keep in mind that a single pound of fat is going to equate to 3,500 calories. So, to put it simply, if you want to lose 1 pound, you need to burn 3,500 calories. If you want to lose 2 pounds, you have to burn 7,000 calories and so on...

So, to compute for your total daily caloric intake, you just have to take your TDEE and decrease it by around 500 to 1,000 depending on how drastic you want your weight loss to be. Of course, the safest and most sustainable caloric deficit for you to take every day would be just 500 to 1,000 calories. However, there are some people who are capable of fast-tracking their weight loss by exceeding that threshold. If you are an experienced fitness enthusiast, maybe you can experiment with going higher. However, if you are just a beginner, try your best to just stay within this range.

If you are consistently generating a deficit of 500 calories per day over the span of a week, then you will have lost at least 1 pound within that same span. So, assuming that you have a TDEE of 2,300 calories and you are looking to lose 1 pound in a week, that means you would have to consume 1,800 calories per day. Take note that your TDEE is going to change as you get slimmer and leaner. So, as a result, you might have to adjust your TDCI values along the way as well.

Step 6: Calculate Your Macros for High- and Low-Carb Days

This is a step that has already been discussed exhaustively in the previous chapter. If you need a quick refresher, feel free to go back and read about it. However, the general rule of thumb here is that you shouldn't try to shoot for anything too far below 100 grams of carbohydrates even on your low-carb days. As a woman, you still need these carbs in order for your body to function healthily and properly. Remember, carb cycling is merely about limiting and managing your carb intake properly. It's not about eliminating carbohydrates altogether.

Also, in addition to that, don't forget to keep in mind that your protein consumption should remain relatively consistent on both your high- and low-carb days. It's typically with your intake of fats and carbs where you get more freedom to play around with. On high-carb days, lessen your consumption of fats. On low-carb days, increase your consumption of fats. And make sure that you're doing all of that while still keeping your total daily caloric intake in mind. If you really want to lose weight on your designated schedule, then you need to stay strict with your daily caloric intake so that you are always able to hit the proper deficit numbers.

Step 7: Figure Out Your Menstrual Cycle Phases

Now, you need to start figuring out where you are on your menstrual cycle. Start plotting your phases. Again, the reason that this is essential for women to do is because your menstrual cycle can really impact the hormone levels of your body. And your capacity to burn fat and lose weight also largely depend on your hormone levels. So, in order for you to maximize your diet and your training, you have to be able to synchronize your health practices with your menstrual cycles appropriately.

Essentially, the first day of your menstrual cycle is the day of your first full blood flow. This cycle should last approximately 28 days. If you have an irregular period, you can always opt to just synchronize your diet with the lunar cycle as it also lasts for the same length of time.

Step 8: Plot Out Your High- and Low-Carb Days

This is a topic that has already been discussed exhaustively in a previous chapter. If you need a refresher on it, feel free to go back. However, for the short form, just remember that you are going to be primed to burn a lot of calories during the first two weeks of your cycle and then your body becomes more sluggish towards the final two weeks. So, you would want to situate more high- or moderate-carb days in the first two weeks. Then, you will want to incorporate more low-carb days in the final two weeks of your cycle.

Also, another general rule of thumb that you want to remember is that on your more active days, you have more liberty to consume carbohydrates. However, on recovery days or times when you don't really exert too much energy, it would be best for you to stick to low carb consumption so as to stay within a caloric deficit.

Step 9: Plan Your Meals Accordingly

At this point, you've already figured out a lot of things. By now, you know that there is some room for improvement with your body, and you have set goals for yourself moving forward. You know how many calories that you burn every day. You are now aware of what kind of caloric deficit you need to achieve and the numbers that you need to hit to achieve them. Because of your dedication to achieving your goals, you have decided that you want to form a workout routine and that you're sticking to it. You've also been oriented about how your menstrual cycles affect how your body processes calories and energy. So, you have developed a plan to sync your diet with your menstrual cycle, and you have all of the calculations planned out.

Now, it's just a matter of you putting real meals into the equation. Remember that all of your macros and your calories are mere numeric representations of the food that you eat. You have finally reached the step where you have to begin researching food and recipes that will help you form your meal plan for the week or even the whole month. If you are in need of some ideas for recipes, then you can refer to the following chapter of this book.

Step 10: Review Your Plan and Make Sure Everything Is Done Right

Lastly, you have to make sure that your plan is rock solid. Again, with carb cycling, half of the battle is done during the planning and preparation phases. If you get a few variables wrong in this initial phase, then you are potentially compromising your entire diet plan as a whole. It's very important that you go over your plan and check the numbers again. See if they all add up.

Also, along the way, feel free to revisit the plan and make a few tweaks here and there whenever you feel like it. A plan isn't designed to last forever. As you lose more weight, your body will undergo certain changes that could affect the variables that were involved in drafting your plan in the first place. With that, it's a good idea for you to revisit your plan every so often just to make sure that you are continuously optimizing your plan for weight loss and fat burn.

Best Food Sources for Carbohydrates

So, we've covered all of the basic reminders that you need to keep to heart while you're developing your plan. You've also been guided on the specific steps that you need to take to develop your carb cycling plan. You're practically set already. You've determined how many calories you need to be eating every day along with all of the macros that make up your calories. At this point, you should also already know when your high-carb and low-carb days should ideally be. Now, it's just a matter of you taking the time to do some research for recipes that you can use to fill up your eating schedule. Don't worry, this book has you covered on that front too. But more on the recipes later. Right now, you might just be thinking about what kind of food you will be eating on your high- and low-carb days.

Okay, there's one common misconception that people get whenever they get into carb cycling diets. You might think that on high-carb days, you have the freedom to drown yourself in bowl after bowl of ice cream. You might assume that it would be okay for you to have as much cake as you want during your high-carb days as long as you stay strict on your low-carb days. True enough, if you crunch the numbers correctly, you might be able to get away with losing weight even when you're eating cake and ice cream all of the time. However, that wouldn't be a holistic approach to overall fitness. Also, it's not sustainable.

There are just certain carb sources that you will want to avoid as much as possible, even during your high-carb days. It's important to stress that while you might be desperate to lose weight, getting leaner isn't always going to be the strongest indicator of overall health and wellness. So, for the purpose of still staying fit and healthy while carb cycling, here is a list of carbs that you need to eat and carbs you need to avoid while dieting.

Carbs to Eat

- bananas
- mangoes
- strawberries
- blueberries
- blackberries
- cherries
- lettuce
- cauliflower
- broccoli
- squash
- tomatoes
- papayas
- bitter gourds
- bean sprouts
- lemons
- avocados
- whole grains
- wheat pasta
- sweet potato
- whole wheat bread
- quinoa
- couscous
- amaranth, etc.

Carbs to Avoid

- white bread
- white rice
- ice cream
- fried potatoes
- refined sugar
- refined flour
- pastries
- cakes
- sugary sauces/dressings
- sodas
- sugary energy drinks
- alcoholic beverages, etc.

If we just keep on listing different kinds of food here, then the book will go on and on. But you get the general picture, right? As much as possible, when choosing your carb sources, try to keep it as fresh and as natural as possible. Go for foods that undergo little to no processing. Stay away from foods that are drenched in sugar or that have undergone substantial processing. Remember that weight loss isn't just a matter of keeping track of your calories. It's also about the quality of the food that you eat. If you eat better, your metabolic system just functions better, and you set yourself up for losing more weight in the future.

Again, take note that the ultimate goal here is health and wellness. Weight loss just plays a vital part of that, but it's not the priority. You can lose all the weight that you want, but if you're just munching on soda and ice cream throughout that period, you're not really healthy.

Final Thoughts

Be proud of yourself for taking that extra step. You've already come up with a rough plan for yourself to help you achieve all of your weight loss goals. Now, it's just a matter of polishing and fine-tuning your plan, and then actually executing it. That might be the scary part for a lot of people, but you shouldn't worry too much. The worst-case scenario is that you end up not achieving your weight loss goals, and you have to do the planning process all over again. That is a heck of a lot better than not even trying at all. However, if you really followed all of the lessons and principles that have been laid out in this book, it's unlikely that you're going to fail at this. Again, all of the tools and foundations are there. You just have to make sure that you are putting them all to good use.

But on the off chance that you do realize that the results just aren't what you're expecting, don't be afraid to go back to the drawing board to start over. There is no shame in going back to the start and finding out where you went wrong. It would be even more shameful if you just continue to stick to a plan that is obviously not working for you or if you just abandon dieting altogether.

Chapter 5:
High- and Low-Carb Recipes

Don't worry. You might already be freaking out if you're someone who isn't very confident about your culinary skills. The recipes that are listed in this book aren't all that complex or difficult. You won't need to undergo years of training in a culinary institute to be able to execute these meals properly. Also, these recipes are mere suggestions. You can always put your own spin on things and simplify them to your own personal preferences. However, these recipes are already pretty simple enough to begin with, so you don't have to worry too much about that.

In this chapter, various recipes will be given to cover the different meals of the day. One of the best aspects of carb cycling is that you don't really have to limit the amount of times that you eat in a day. It's merely a matter of controlling portion sizes. So, if you play your cards right, you can have three full meals plus a snack every day without worrying about getting fat or gaining weight. Also, aside from teaching you how to execute these meals in this kitchen, these recipes also come with serving size suggestions together with corresponding nutritional information. You will be given the values for macros and calories with these recipes so that you have a better idea of how you can insert these meals into your overall meal plan.

Again, don't be afraid of getting creative with these. After all, it's you who is going to be eating these meals in the end. Just know that any changes you make to the recipes might also result in changes of the numerical values of the nutritional info. With that said, here are some recipes for high- and low-carb meals that you can incorporate into your carb cycling plan.

Breakfast

4-Egg and Cheese Omelette with Toast Slices (Low Carb)

Servings: 1

Preparation Time: 5 minutes

Cook Time: 5 minutes

Ingredients:

- 1 tbsp olive oil
- 4 medium-sized eggs
- 1 ½ oz of cheese
- 2 slices of whole wheat bread
- salt and pepper to taste

Instructions:

1. Prepare a skillet and place it over medium heat and add olive oil.

2. Brush olive oil all around the skillet and allow to heat up.

3. While skillet is heating up, crack the four eggs into a large bowl and whisk thoroughly with a fork or eggbeater.

4. Then, add the eggs to the skillet and stir continuously as it cooks. Make sure to never stop stirring to prevent the eggs from becoming rubbery or tough.

5. Once the eggs are cooked, turn off the heat, and add the cheese to the eggs. Continue to stir to fully incorporate the cheese into the eggs.

6. Set the eggs on a plate and serve together with two slices of wheat bread.

7. Season the eggs with salt and pepper to taste.

Nutritional Information:

Calories: 383 kcal, Carbs: 36 g, Fat: 17 g, Protein: 21 g

Cream Cheese Pancakes (Low Carb)

Servings: 1

Preparation Time: 3 minutes

Cook Time: 9 minutes

Ingredients:

- 2 oz of cream cheese

- 2 eggs

- 1 tsp of low carb sweetener

- ½ tsp cinnamon powder

Instructions:

1. Prepare a high-power blender and add all of the ingredients.

2. Blend it all together on high until it achieves a smooth and thick consistency.

3. Allow to rest for 2 minutes so that the bubbles will settle.

4. Prepare a non-stick skillet and place it over medium heat.

5. Grease the pan with butter or non-stick spray.

6. Once the pan is hot, add ¼ of the batter to the pan in a clean circular shape.

7. Cook for two minutes or until it achieves a golden-brown color on the bottom.

8. Flip the pancake and allow the other side to cook for another minute.

9. Repeat this process until you run out of batter.

10. (Optional) Serve with low-carb syrup or berries as toppings.

Nutritional Information:

Calories: 344 kcal, Carbs: 3 g, Fat: 29 g, Protein: 17 g

Keto Coconut Porridge (Low Carb)

Servings: 1

Preparation Time: 5 minutes

Cook Time: 5 minutes

Ingredients:

- 1 large egg
- 1 tbsp of coconut flour
- 1 pinch of ground psyllium husk powder
- 1 oz butter (room temperature)
- 4 tbsp of coconut cream
- salt to taste

Instructions:

1. In a medium-sized bowl, add the egg and whisk until thoroughly beaten.

2. Then, add the coconut flour, psyllium husk powder, and salt to the mixture.

3. Prepare a small pan and place it over low heat. Melt the butter and coconut cream in the pan. Make sure that both ingredients are well incorporated.

4. Gradually add the egg mixture into the pan and mix thoroughly until you achieve a thick and creamy texture.

5. (Optional) Top your porridge with berries, nuts, or coconut shavings.

Nutritional Information:

Calories: 486 kcal, Carbs: 4 g, Fat: 49 g, Protein: 9 g

Fruity Oatmeal Bowl (High Carb)

Servings: 2

Preparation Time: 5 minutes

Cook Time: 5 minutes

Ingredients:

- 1 cup rolled oats
- natural sweeteners to taste (like honey)
- ¼ cup coconut milk
- 1 banana (sliced)
- ½ mango (peeled and thinly sliced)
- 1 kiwi (peeled and sliced)
- ¼ cup pineapple (diced)
- 2 tbsp raspberries
- 1 tbsp coconut flakes

Instructions:

1. Cook the oatmeal as directed on the package instructions.
2. Stir the coconut milk into the pot of oatmeal and add your desired amount of sweetener.
3. Incorporate the fruits into the oatmeal and garnish with coconut flakes.
4. Serve either chilled or warm.

Nutritional Information:

Calories: 348 kcal, Carbs: 59 g, Fat: 10 g, Protein:7 g

Lunch

Zucchini and Walnut Salad (Low Carb)

Servings: 4

Preparation Time: 5 minutes

Cook Time: 2 minutes

Ingredients:

For the Dressing:

- 2 tbsp olive oil
- ¾ cup mayonnaise
- 2 tsp lemon juice
- 1 clove of garlic (minced)
- ½ tsp salt
- ¼ tsp chili powder

For the Salad:

- 1 head of romaine lettuce
- 4 oz of arugula
- ¼ cup of chopped scallions
- 2 whole zucchinis
- 1 tbsp olive oil
- 3 ½ oz of chopped walnuts
- salt and pepper to taste

Instructions:

1. Prepare a small bowl and add all of the ingredients for the dressing.

2. Incorporate all of the dressing ingredients well and set aside.

3. In a large bowl, combine the trimmed romaine, arugula, and chives. Make sure that all of the ingredients are mixed well.

4. On a cutting board, split both zucchinis lengthwise and remove the seeds. Then, cut the zucchinis into small half-inch pieces crosswise.

5. Prepare a medium-sized skillet and place it over medium heat. Add olive oil to the pan and allow to heat until it shimmers. Then, add the zucchini pieces to the skillet and season with salt and pepper.

6. Allow the zucchini to cook until slightly browned on the outside. Then, add the nuts to the pan and cook both ingredients together.

7. Add the zucchini and the walnuts to the lettuce leaves and then drizzle with salad dressing.

Nutritional Information:

Calories: 595 kcal, Carbs: 8 g, Fat: 58 g, Protein: 9 g

Salad in a Jar (Low Carb)

Servings: 1

Preparation Time: 5 minutes

Cook Time: N/A

Ingredients:

- 1 oz of romaine lettuce
- ½ scallion
- 1 carrot
- 1 avocado
- 1 oz cherry tomatoes
- 1 oz red bell peppers
- 4 oz smoked salmon
- ¼ cup mayonnaise

Instructions:

1. Shred and chop all of the vegetables into reasonably small portions.

2. When assembling the salad in the jar, place the green and leafy vegetables at the bottom to serve as the base.

3. Add the other ingredients in their own respective layers.

4. Top the salad with the smoked salmon.

5. Add your dressing just before serving.

Nutritional Information:

Calories: 876 kcal, Carbs: 11 g, Fat: 76 g, Protein: 27 g

Moroccan Couscous with Flank Steak
(High Carb)

Servings: 5

Preparation Time: 5 minutes

Cook Time: 10 minutes

Ingredients:

- 1 ¼ lb lean flank steak (chopped into 1-inch cubes)
- 1 tbsp olive oil
- 1 cup red onion (diced)
- 1 red bell pepper (diced)
- 1 ½ tbsp minced garlic
- ⅔ cup frozen peas
- ⅔ cup shredded carrots
- 1 ½ cup low-sodium beef broth
- 1 cup dry couscous
- 2 tbsp fresh mint
- ⅓ cup raisins
- 2 tsp smoked paprika
- 1 tsp cumin
- 1 tsp turmeric
- ½ tsp cayenne powder
- 1 tsp coriander
- ½ tsp cinnamon

Instructions:

1. Prepare a non-stick skillet and set it on high heat. Brush or spray the skillet with oil or non-stick spray and then add the beef cubes. Season the beef with salt and pepper. Allow the beef to sear on one side for one minute before shaking the pan to sear the other sides. Cook the beef until you've achieved your desired readiness and then remove it from the skillet.

2. Lower the heat to medium and add olive oil, garlic, salt, onions, bell pepper, and black pepper. Cook for around 2 minutes or until the onions become slightly translucent. Add all of the powder spices to the pan and make sure that the onions and bell peppers are seasoned properly.

3. Add the frozen peas and carrots to the pan, and then immediately pour in the beef broth.

4. Bring the broth to a light simmer and add the couscous. Gently incorporate everything together inside of the broth and remove from the heat to allow the couscous to absorb the liquid. This should take no more than 5 minutes.

5. Mix in the beef and serve in equal portions.

Nutritional Information:

Calories: 371 kcal, Carbs: 41 g, Fat: 9 g, Protein: 32 g

Slow-Cooked Chicken and Rice Casserole
(High Carb)

Servings: 5

Preparation Time: 10 minutes

Cook Time: 4 hours

Ingredients:

- 1 lb chicken breast (chopped into 1-inch pieces)
- 3 ½ cups low-sodium chicken broth
- 1 cup uncooked brown rice
- ½ cup 2% Greek yogurt
- ⅔ cup cheddar cheese
- 12 oz raw broccoli florets
- 1 tbsp olive oil
- 1 tbsp garlic (minced)
- ½ red onion (diced)
- 1 tsp thyme
- 1 tsp rosemary

Instructions:

1. Prepare a slow cooker and set it to a sauté function on low heat. Add the olive oil, onions, and garlic into the slow cooker until the onions are caramelized. This should take around 3 to 5 minutes.

2. Add the brown rice, thyme, and rosemary. Make sure that the spices are well incorporated into the brown rice.

3. Pour the chicken broth into the cooker and follow it with the raw chicken breasts. Cook the rice and chicken for around 3 to 5 hours.

4. When there's around 30 minutes to 1 hour left of cooking, stir the Greek yogurt and cheese into the slow cooker. Mix everything until the liquid becomes thick and creamy.

5. Place the raw broccoli on top of the rice, but do not mix it. Allow the heat to soften the broccoli.

6. Allow the entire meal to cook for the remaining time.

7. Season with salt and pepper and serve.

Nutritional Information:

Calories: 380 kcal, Carbs: 36 g, Fat: 11 g, Protein: 36 g

Dinner

Turkey Sandwich on Whole Wheat (Low Carb)

Servings: 1

Preparation Time: 20 minutes

Cook Time: N/A

Ingredients:

- 1 large lettuce head
- 2 slices of whole wheat bread
- 1 tsp of cream cheese
- ¼ red onion
- ¼ small cucumber (slices)
- 25 grams of sprouts
- 31 grams of sliced turkey ham (lean)
- salt and pepper to taste

Instructions:

1. Remove the lettuce leaves from the head and rinse thoroughly. Set the leaves aside and allow to dry.

2. While waiting for the leaves to dry, prepare the two slices of bread and spread the cream cheese evenly along the surface of one slice.

3. Take the cucumber and rinse thoroughly. Then, slice it into very thin portions.

4. Peel the onion and then rinse it thoroughly. Thinly slice the onion into rings.

5. Prepare the sprouts and rinse them thoroughly. Shake them to remove any excess water and allow to dry for a bit.

6. On a serving plate or cutting board, place the slice of bread without cream cheese on the bottom to serve as the base of the sandwich. Then, add the lettuce leaves and season with salt and pepper. After that, proceed to add layers of ham, onions, cucumbers, and sprouts. Lightly season each layer along the way.

7. Top the sandwich with the remaining slice of bread and serve as is.

Nutritional Information:

Calories: 241 kcal, Carbs: 36 g, Fat: 4.5 g, Protein: 15.5 g

Fried Kale and Broccoli Salad (Low Carb)

Servings: 2

Preparation Time: 5 minutes

Cook Time: 10 to 12 minutes

Ingredients:

- ½ cup mayonnaise
- 1 tbsp whole-grain mustard
- 4 eggs
- ½ lb broccoli
- 4 oz of kale
- 2 scallions
- 2 garlic cloves
- 2 avocados
- 2 tbsp olive oil
- chili flakes, salt, and pepper to taste

Instructions:

1. Add water to a large pot and fill it up halfway. Submerge the unpeeled eggs into the pot of water and place the pot over medium heat. Bring the water to a light boil and allow the eggs to cook for 8 to 10 minutes.

2. While the eggs are cooking, prepare a large bowl of ice and water to serve as an ice bath for the eggs.

3. In a separate small bowl, mix the mayo and mustard together and set aside.

4. Once cooked, remove the eggs from the pot and place the eggs in the ice bath prior to peeling.

5. Once the eggs have cooled, peel them and slice them into halves or quarters.

6. Split the avocados in half. Remove the pits and cut the meat into slices.

7. Slice the cloves of garlic as thinly as you can and fry them up over a hot skillet with olive oil. Cook the garlic until they are crispy and set aside on top of a paper towel.

8. Chop the kale and broccoli coarsely and cook in the frying pan together with butter. Fry the vegetables over medium-high heat until they have softened.

9. Add the kale and broccoli to a large bowl with avocados, eggs, and the mayo-mustard dressing. Season everything with salt, chili flakes, and pepper. Top it with crunchy garlic slices and serve.

Nutritional Information:

Calories: 1022 kcal, Carbs: 13 g, Fat: 94 g, Protein: 22 g

Sweet and Spicy Beef Bowl (High Carb)

Servings: 4

Preparation Time: 5 minutes

Cook Time: 15 minutes

Ingredients:

- 12 oz sugar snap peas
- 2 radicchio (chopped)
- juice from ½ lemon
- 2 cups of cooked brown rice
- 1 ½ lb flank steak (chopped into ½ inch cubes)

For the sauce:

- 3 tbsp low-sodium soy sauce
- 2 tbsp fresh ginger
- 2 tsp sesame oil
- 2 tbsp water
- 3 tbsp sriracha
- 4 tbsp coconut sugar
- juice from one whole orange
- 1 ½ tbsp arrowroot starch

For garnish:

- orange wedge
- sesame seeds
- chopped scallions

Instructions:

1. Mix together all of the ingredients for the sauce except for the arrowroot. Set the sauce and the arrowroot aside for the meantime.

2. Prepare a large non-stick pan and set it over high heat. Once the pan has heated, add the sugar peas first and cook until soft. Make sure to continuously stir the peas so as to prevent charring on the outside. This should take around 3 minutes.

3. Remove the peas from the skillet once they are cooked. Then, add the radicchio to the pan. While the radicchio is cooking, add some lemon juice. Continue to cook until the radicchio begins to wilt. Once cooked, remove the radicchio from the pan.

4. Then, add the chopped beef into the pan and sear until it has achieved your desired readiness. Once the beef is cooked, reduce the heat of the pan and move the beef towards the sides, creating a big gap in the middle.

5. Add the arrowroot to your sauce and add the entire sauce mixture to the center of the skillet. Once the sauce begins to bubble or thicken, remove the pan from the heat and continuously fold the beef into the sauce.

6. Remove the beef from the pan and garnish with scallions and sesame seeds.

7. Add the beef on top of the brown rice and mix together with radicchio and sugar snap peas.

8. Divide into equal portions and serve.

Nutritional Information:

Calories: 459 kcal, Carbs: 45 g, Fat: 11 g, Protein: 40 g

Spicy Avocado Chicken Salad Wrap

Servings: 1

Preparation Time: 5 minutes

Cook Time: 5 minutes

Ingredients:

- 1 large whole wheat tortilla
- 4 oz cooked chicken breast (chopped)
- 1 ½ cups of chopped romaine lettuce
- ½ beefsteak tomato (chopped)
- ⅓ cup cucumber (chopped)
- ½ medium avocado (chopped)
- ¾ tbsp Cajun seasoning powder
- 2 tbsp plain yogurt

Instructions:

1. Place the chicken in a large bowl and season with the Cajun powder. Make sure that the chicken is well coated with the seasoning.

2. Add the rest of the ingredients into the bowl except for the tortilla.

3. Mix the contents of the bowl thoroughly with a spatula until they are all well incorporated.

4. Take the tortilla and warm it in the microwave for around 10 to 15 seconds. Take the tortilla out of the microwave and place it on a flat, stable surface.

5. Add the salad mix to the center of the tortilla and fold the sides together. Roll the entire tortilla until it forms a burrito.

6. Serve the burrito sliced or whole.

Nutritional Information:

Calories: 534 kcal, Carbs: 49 g, Fat: 18 g, Protein: 47 g

Snacks

Almond Milkshake (Low Carb)

Servings: 1

Preparation Time: 5 minutes

Cook Time: N/A

Ingredients:

- 1 oz of almonds
- 1 cup of full-cream milk
- 1 cup of ice cubes
- zero-calorie sweetener (Stevia, Splenda, etc.)

Instructions:

1. Add the ice cubes to a high-power blender and set it to crush.
2. Crush the ice until it achieves a snowy consistency.
3. Add the full-cream milk and the almonds to the blender and set it to blend.
4. Blend the ingredients until they are all well incorporated with one another.
5. (Optional) Add sweetener to the mixture and serve chilled.

Nutritional Information:

Calories: 264 kcal, Carbs: 20 g, Fat: 16 g, Protein: 14 g

Low-Carb Deviled Eggs (Low Carb)

Servings: 4

Preparation Time: 5 minutes

Cook Time: 12 minutes

Ingredients:

- 4 large eggs
- ¼ cup mayonnaise
- 1 tsp tabasco
- 8 strips of smoked salmon
- fresh dill and salt to taste

Instructions:

1. Add water to a large pot and fill it up halfway. Submerge the unpeeled eggs into the pot of water and place the pot over medium heat. Bring the water to a light boil and allow the eggs to cook for 8 to 10 minutes.

2. While the eggs are cooking, prepare a large bowl of ice and water to serve as an ice bath for the eggs.

3. Once cooked, remove the eggs from the pot and place the eggs in the ice bath prior to peeling.

4. Once the eggs have cooled, remove the shells and split the eggs in half. Scoop the yolk out of the eggs and place the yolks and whites on separate plates.

5. Mash the egg yolks with a masher or a fork and add salt, mayonnaise, and tabasco.

6. Once all of the ingredients in the egg yolk mixture are well incorporated, add them back to the egg whites and top with a small strip of smoked salmon.

7. Decorate each egg with dill and serve.

Nutritional Information:

Calories: 163 kcal, Carbs: 0.5 g, Fat: 15 g, Protein: 7 g

Peanut Butter Sandwich on Wheat Bread (High Carb)

Servings: 1

Preparation Time: 2 minutes

Cook Time: N/A

Ingredients:

- 2 tbsp of peanut butter
- 2 slices of whole wheat bread

Instructions:

1. Prepare the two slices of bread and arrange each slice on a stable surface.

2. Spread one tablespoon of peanut butter on each slice of bread.

3. Combine both slices together or eat them independently.

4. (Optional) Place the sandwich on top of a hot skillet and allow to cook for one minute on each side to make the bread crunchier.

Nutritional Information:

Calories: 327 kcal, Carbs: 30 g, Fat: 18 g, Protein: 15 g

Multigrain Bread with Olive Oil

Servings: 1

Preparation Time: 2 minutes

Cook Time: N/A

Ingredients:

- 1 tbsp olive oil
- 2 slices of multigrain bread
- salt to taste

Instructions:

1. Lightly toast multigrain bread in a toaster or on top of skillet.

2. Pour olive oil into a small dipping bowl and add salt to taste.

3. Break bread apart with hands and dip into olive oil prior to eating.

Nutritional Information:

Calories: 257 kcal, Carbs: 22.6 g, Fat: 16.2 g, Protein: 7 g

Chapter 6:
Tips and Tricks for Success

At this point, you should already have everything that you need to start your carb cycling diet plan. However, the book isn't over yet. We're not going to leave you hanging just yet. Just because you have everything that you need doesn't mean that you still won't stand to benefit from learning a few of the tips and tricks of the trade. Again, the road to success in weight loss and fitness isn't going to be without its fair share of bumps and hitches. You are bound to make a few mistakes here and there, but that's okay. That's a part of the process.

However, there are a few ways that you can minimize your chances of making mistakes. Here are a few tips and tricks that you can keep up your sleeve just to make sure that you are putting yourself in the best possible position to succeed.

Drink Lots of Water

For the very first tip, you need to make it a point to always hydrate. Water is life... quite literally. Did you know that water makes up 60% of your body? That fact alone should serve as enough incentive for you to up your water intake. When you drink lots of water, you are constantly hydrating your muscles and your vital organs. This means that your body is going to be able to function more efficiently for metabolizing food and for working out as well.

On top of that, water can also help curb hunger. A lot of the time, when people think that they're hungry, they're really just thirsty. So, the next time you think you're craving that fried chicken sandwich, reach for a glass of water instead. You will be surprised at how often you will be able to curb your cravings just by drinking a glass of water. Make sure that you always have a bottle or glass of water near you at all times. This way, it's much easier for you to always keep yourself hydrated.

Set Concrete and Realistic Goals

Goal setting is always going to be important in whatever endeavor you choose to engage in. Sure, when you're just starting out, it's so easy to set goals like *"I want to be healthier,"* or *"I want to lose a lot of weight,"* and that's fine. These are valid goals to have. However, when you're just starting out, it's important that you set goals that are more concrete and less ambiguous. Of course, you want to lose a lot of weight. But it would be better to attribute a specific number to that particular goal.

So, instead of saying that you want to lose an arbitrary amount of weight, put a real number to it. Say you want to lose 5 pounds next month. Say you want to lose 2 pounds this week. When you are shooting for concrete and realistic goals like this, it becomes a lot easier to track your progress. And it doesn't even just have to be about your weight. Here are a few examples of goals that you can set for yourself:

- I want to go five straight days without cheating on my diet.
- I want to be able to run 5 km in under 30 minutes.
- I want to fit back into my old pair of jeans.
- I want to wake up at 6 a.m. every day to work out.

When you have more specific and concrete goals like this, the whole process becomes a lot easier to absorb and digest.

Don't Pay Too Much Attention to the Scale

Okay, it's important to stress this point, especially since we've talked about setting more concrete goals for yourself. Yes, in the previous tip, you were advised to be more concrete about how much weight you want to lose. So, that means that you need to check your weight consistently to know if you're making progress. That's the right idea. However, too many people make the mistake of obsessing over the number that is on the scale. Keep in mind that weight loss is not a linear process. Your weight is going to keep on fluctuating. You will lose weight and you will gain it back. That's just the nature of weight loss.

So, if you keep on obsessing over the number that's on the scale, you might end up thinking that you're doing things wrong even though you're doing everything right. Instead of checking the scales every day, try doing so just once a week or every two weeks instead. Also, the scale only tells half the story. Remember that muscles are heavier than fats. So, if you're burning fat and you're gaining muscle, you might not be losing that much weight. But if that's the case, your body fat percentage is still going down and that's the ultimate goal. Also, another better indicator of true weight loss is checking your waistline. Sometimes, the number on the scale might not be going down so much. But if your waistline is getting smaller, that's a better indicator of more effective weight loss.

Do Meal Planning and Preparation

There's a reason why multiple chapters in this book have been dedicated to you really planning and preparing your meals in advance. Okay, there are two aspects of this tip. There is the planning aspect and there is the preparation aspect. Both aspects are equally important, and you really need to incorporate both habits into your life of health and wellness.

First, planning. With carb cycling, it's not just a matter of you deciding on the spot whether you will have a high- or low-carb day. You aren't going to find much success with this diet if you're going to go about it whimsically. You need to consciously plan your low- and high-carb days as you consider other factors of your lifestyle like training schedule, training intensity, and menstrual cycle. The old adage says that a failure to plan is a plan to fail. So, don't disregard the whole planning process of carb cycling.

Next, there is meal preparation. This tip is all about practicality. When you engage in meal planning, then you know all of the food that you're going to consume over an extended period. Since you already have that knowledge, it would also be best for you to prepare most of your meals in advance as well. This is going to save you the trouble of having to cook food up every single time you want to eat. Part of being able to stick to a diet is having healthy food readily available at any moment's notice. Most people find success in bulk cooking. They take one day out of every week, and they dedicate it to preparing ALL of the meals for that week. Of course, you can stagger your meals so that they're not always repetitive. It's all up to you.

Remember Fat Isn't the Enemy

Contrary to what many people believe, fat is actually not the enemy. Eating fat isn't going to make you fat. Again, this is a point that has already been proven time and time again by practitioners of the keto diet. Just because you're eating a lot of fat doesn't necessarily mean that that food is going to be processed into fat for your body. The real enemy here is sugar. Remember that sugar is what is converted into glucose and is used as energy for your body. However, if you eat too much sugar, a lot of that glucose doesn't get used up, and it gets converted into stored fat in the body.

Also, the thing about sugar is that it's so addictive and easy to consume. It can be so easy to go overboard on the calories from mere sugar consumption. This is why a diet plan like carb cycling, which directly manages and oversees the healthy consumption of carbohydrates and sugar, is so effective. Instead of vilifying fat, it would be better to demonize empty carbs like sugar instead.

Stick to a Solid Workout Plan

Training shouldn't be sporadic either. Again, with this kind of diet, it's really going to be at its most effective state if you pair it with a healthy training regimen. And when we say healthy training regimen, we're talking about an actual plan that you can stick to over a prolonged period. It's not enough that you decide to run a 5k today, rest a few days, and then join a yoga class when you feel like you have the energy. That's not what a workout plan is.

This is why goal setting is so important in fitness. For instance, if you make it a concrete goal for yourself to run a half-marathon in six months, then that means that you have to follow a strict running program for you to stay in shape. Maybe, if you make it a goal to attend five yoga classes per week, then that means you have a solid plan for yourself in terms of scheduling. Also, keep in mind that your low- and high-carb days are going to be dependent on what kind of workout plan you have. Again, this isn't just something that you can approach whimsically and expect to yield positive results.

Cook Your Own Meals

So, what is the best way for you to really know how much food you're eating? It's when you take the time to really measure and cook your own meals. Sure, you can always opt to go for the easier route by going to restaurants and ordering meals from there. However, what is easy isn't always going to be the most accurate. There's no way you can really gauge the macros and calories in a meal that you order from a restaurant because you weren't there during the cooking and preparation process.

Of course, there are also various healthy meal service providers out there who offer calorie-counted options for you. You can always opt to go that route as well. However, these services tend to be very pricey, and it might not be the practical thing for most people. This should only serve as the last resort when you don't think that you have the time or the skills to cook delicious, healthy meals for yourself. However, ultimately, anyone can cook to a certain degree. A lot of the recipes listed in this book are designed for beginners and novices in the kitchen. It's just a matter of taking the time to really master cooking these recipes.

Avoid Drinking Calories

Much to the dismay of many people, calories also exist in drinks. Yes. The one or two glasses of wine that you have after dinner are also going to bring calories with them as well. That bottle of Gatorade or Red Bull that you drank to fuel your workout? Those have calories in them as well. The thing about beverages like these is that they are incredibly deceptive. They pack a lot of calories, but they don't really do much good for the body from a nutrition standpoint. So, as much as possible just stick to water.

Of course, there are some beverages out there that have little to no calories at all like tea or coffee. Things only get dangerous when you start adding sweeteners or creamers to these beverages. If you must have a beverage other than water, you can always opt for tea or coffee. Also, the caffeine content of these beverages is known to help improve your metabolism and facilitate fat burn. Just make sure that you don't go overboard with adding artificial or natural sweeteners and creamers. It would be much better if you get your calories from whole foods like lean proteins or whole grains.

Don't Go Grocery Shopping While Hungry or Without a Plan

This tip might seem rather silly, but there's actually real scientific backing to it. Whenever you are hungry, it's known that you don't really have the ability to think at your logical peak. This is because your mind is distracted, and it can't really focus on the tasks that it must accomplish. It's the same with grocery shopping too. You might think that it's such a menial task that it doesn't require much focus or logic. However, this is where you would be wrong.

If you go into a grocery store while you're hungry, your mind will trick itself into thinking that you should be buying things that you don't really need. Ideally, you will go into a grocery store with a set grocery list and just stick to that. You won't choose things on a whim. You might end up buying a lot of unnecessary or unhealthy food items that could potentially compromise your diet. So, the best course of action will be for you to fill yourself up before visiting the grocery store. And make sure that you have a grocery list ready. Stick to that list!

Evolve Your Goals Along the Way

Earlier in this list, you were taught that you need to really be serious about setting your goals before you embark on your fitness journey. However, please know that your goals are never set in stone and that they are subject to occasional changes and evolution. Again, as you become fitter and leaner, your body is going to undergo some very significant changes. These changes are all for the better, of course. However, that also means that a lot of the goals that you set at the start might become obsolete. This is why it's essential that you continuously evolve your goals along the way.

For instance, if you had your sights set on losing 10 pounds in one month originally, perhaps you can taper it down to 7 or 8 pounds in the next month. Your body is going to find it difficult to burn more fat the leaner it gets. So, it would be smart for you to taper your weight loss goals gradually as you go. Another example is if you make it a goal to run a half-marathon. Naturally, if you complete that goal, then you might want to evolve and aim for running a full marathon. If you constantly evolve your goals, then you will realize the work is never done. In this sense, you keep pushing for self-improvement and development.

Don't Give Up on a Diet Too Quickly

This is a common mistake that a lot of people make whenever they're just starting out. Keep in mind that everyone's body is going to function differently. This means that not all people are going to yield the same results or responses towards a certain diet. Just because you have a friend who lost weight in two weeks from carb cycling doesn't mean that it's going to be the same for you. Sometimes, the effects take much longer for other people. There are a variety of factors to consider here such as genetics, lifestyle, and hormones. Ultimately, you will only really be able to see the effects of a diet after at least three to four weeks of strict dieting. If you cheat along the way, then the results might be delayed even further.

Just stick to it. Make sure that you are staying strict with your diet for at least three to four weeks. Don't have any cheat days and see if there are results. If it doesn't work for you, then maybe the plan was off to begin with. Try to make a few adjustments and lower the caloric values for your consumption a bit. If it still doesn't work, then maybe it just isn't a good fit. And that's okay. There's no shame in that. It will only be a waste if you abandon the diet too quickly without ever giving it a chance.

Find Yourself a Diet or Training Buddy

Like love, fitness is something that is best when shared. Of course, you are perfectly capable of achieving all of your goals and dreams on your own. You don't have to be reliant on anyone else to help you achieve your fitness goals. No one is going to do the work for you, and so, no one should ever get to tell you that you can't do something. However, it always helps whenever you have a strong support system. So, if you can recruit a few friends or buddies to help keep you accountable to your goals and duties, then that's good.

Again, it's important to emphasize that you can do everything on your own. But if you have an opportunity to gain the help and support of other people, that is always a plus. You can keep each other honest, and you can celebrate each other's victories. Also, there is this understated energy that you can get from knowing that other people are invested in your success as well. It's a lot more comforting to face a tough journey knowing that you have other people at your side who are willing to help you out.

Stick to Workouts or Diets You Really Enjoy

If you don't have fun doing it, then it's not worth doing. Of course, if you had the choice, in an ideal world, you would be able to eat anything that you want without having to worry about getting fat. Unfortunately, this is not the world that we live in. So, you have to abide by certain fitness rules and principles if you want to remain healthy. However, just because you need to abide by these rules doesn't mean that you won't get the opportunity to have fun in the process. It's important that in your health and fitness journey, you still enjoy what you're doing.

When you're choosing a workout program, it should be physically strenuous enough so you're achieving results. However, it should also be an enjoyable experience for you so that it becomes more sustainable. When selecting a diet program, it has to be strict in the sense that you are adhering to proper nutritional principles. However, it shouldn't be a diet that makes you sad and depressed about life. You should still have a pretty positive and healthy relationship with your food. This is why a flexible diet like carb cycling just works so well for a lot of people. It's not as restrictive as other diets, but it still instills a sense of discipline.

Schedule Your Cheat Days

Okay, this might seem like it's counterintuitive, but there is some logic behind this. As much as possible, you won't want to have any cheat days ever. If it's possible for you to stay strict on your diet forever, then that's a good thing. However, to be quite frank about it, a vast majority of people don't have that kind of willpower. Occasionally, we are going to be entitled to a cheat day and that's okay. Life is meant to be enjoyed, after all. It's all just a matter of keeping things in moderation.

Having said that, it is better if you actually schedule your cheat days instead of just deciding on the spot that you're going to cheat. For example, some people find it effective to stay very strict from Monday to Saturday and then have their cheat days on Sunday. Other people would find it more effective to have one cheat day every two weeks or even just once every month. It all depends. Just make sure that your cheat days aren't getting in the way of your progress. If you have this kind of system in place, you are more motivated to stay strict on the days that you're supposed to be strict.

Get Better Sleep at Night

Lastly, it's very important that you get proper sleep at night. Your sleeping patterns can dramatically impact the way that your body functions. You might not know this, but having poor sleeping patterns can actually impair your metabolic system and result in you retaining more weight. Lacking sleep can result in lower insulin sensitivity, and so your body starts to retain more fat instead of burning more of it. Also, in addition to that, when you lack sleep, you just lack that energy to go work out and be active. Sleep is vital to a body's recovery and rejuvenation. When you don't get to sleep properly at night, your body doesn't get the chance to recuperate the way that it's supposed to. And this can negatively affect athletic performance.

Final Thoughts

Of course, these are only a few tips and tricks that you can use on your own fitness journey. You can choose whether or not to adopt them in your own life. You may also opt to develop your own systems. The only thing that matters here is that you find something that works best for you. It's ultimately about what you can yield from your own personal journey.

A lot of people don't realize that their fitness journeys are also deeply personal ones. A lot of your success is dependent on the kind of relationship that you have with your body, training regimen, and food. And like in real life relationships, there are some relationships that are healthy and there are others that are toxic. Make sure that all of your relationships are wholesome and positive. This way, you always know that you are feeding more positivity into your life and your daily habits.

Author's Note

We're nearing the end of this book, and it's been such an amazing journey. Hopefully, you will have come to learn a lot of things about the way that your body works and what you can do to make the most out of the body that you've been given. If you feel like you have had a great experience with reading this book, please do take the time to leave a short review on Amazon.

Reviews are really not easy to come by. And as an independent author who is working on a small budget, I have to rely on people like you to leave short and honest reviews of my work on Amazon. These reviews serve as the lifeline for my career. I genuinely still want to be of help to many people out there and I need your reviews to keep me afloat. It could even just be a simple sentence or two. I don't want it to be too much of a bother for you.

With that said, I am grateful for you taking the time to read this book in its entirety. It's very heartwarming to know that you were patient enough to heed my advice on this matter. All the best to you and I wish you well on your road to fitness!

Conclusion

There you have it. Those are all of the essentials of learning about carb cycling for women. First of all, congratulations to you for deciding that you still have room for learning and development when it comes to health and wellness. That is always going to be an important first step. It's always essential that people realize that they don't know everything when it comes to their bodies. It takes great humility to pick up a book like this and acknowledge that there is so much left to learn about the ways that our bodies work.

Yes, it's true that the state of obesity in the world can be very saddening and alarming. There are so many people who have been gravely affected by obesity and all its mistresses. People have found the quality of their own lives severely compromised because of their poor eating habits and unhealthy lifestyles. Loads of individuals all over the world have lost their loved ones as a result of diseases or illnesses brought about by obesity. It really is one of the world's greatest killers, and we all need to fight back against it.

Of course, this book isn't saying that carb cycling is *the way* to go for *everyone* in the world. Again, we all find success in many different paths and methodologies. There is no one ideal diet that is best for everyone to follow. There are certain strengths and caveats to each of them. The only proper answer to what the best diet in the world is, is the one that works best for you. It's that simple. So, if you are someone who has managed to find a large degree of success through carb cycling, then that's good. Try to stick with it and be consistent. However, if it doesn't work for you, then that's okay too. The point here is that you are trying and that you're making an effort to improve your own personal health. By doing so, you are also uplifting the state of health and wellness all over the world in your own little way.

Getting fit and healthy isn't the easiest thing to do. Heck, if it were so easy, then everyone in the world would be fit and healthy, right? This is why it's even more important for people like you to really be more conscious about the little habits and routines that you incorporate into your daily life. Earlier in this book, it was mentioned that in order for you to find success, you need to live a life that is more purposeful and structured. That's really the truth, especially when it comes to health and wellness. If you do something that doesn't really add value or serve a purpose to your life, then you are just wasting energy. If you are putting forth unstructured efforts that are inconsistent, then you are wasting energy. One of the greatest keys to being consistent with your success in your health and fitness journey is adding a sense of structure and purpose.

Through it all, there will be various books, articles, journals, and other forms of media out there telling you that their recommended path for fitness is better and more effective. That might actually be true for some people. And it might even be true for you. Never be afraid of learning. Always be willing to open yourself up to opportunities for growth and development, especially in your fitness. If you have an opportunity to learn about a better practice for your health and wellness, then you should capitalize on it.

At the end of the day, it should be your responsibility to yourself to always try to keep up to date on the current and relevant information surrounding physical fitness. It would be an awful waste if you just completely disregard your body and take it for granted. As the old cliché goes, your body is a temple. You should always do your part in making sure that it is cared for.

Even if you have all sorts of problems going on in your life, you can always control how you treat your body. This is a truth that is consistent with everyone. You might be faced with a lot of uncontrollable circumstances, but you can always control how your body chooses to respond to those circumstances. Truthfully, if you take the time to consciously be healthier and fitter, you will find that everything in life just becomes a lot easier. You get a lot more energy and you feel more motivated to do more things. There's a reason why they say that exercise is a natural drug. The rush of endorphins will give you the natural high that you need to really enjoy the life that you've been given.

So, don't throw away your opportunity at living your best life. Regardless if it's with carb cycling or not, just make an effort to be fitter and healthier. You will only thank yourself in the long run for doing so. Fight to be a healthier you. Fight to live in a fitter society. Fight to be a part of a healthier world.

References

Collova, A. (2019, November 2). *IIFYM (If it fits your macros).* https://www.iifym.com/iifym-calculator/iifym-carb-cycling/

GBD 2017 Diet Collaborators. (2019, April 3). Health effects of dietary risks in 195 countries, 1990–2017: a systematic analysis for the Global Burden of Disease Study 2017. Retrieved from https://secure.jbs.elsevierhealth.com/action/cookieAbsent?code=null#%20

Family Health Team. (2019, August 13). *What to eat if you're carb cycling.* https://health.clevelandclinic.org/what-to-eat-if-youre-carb-cycling/

Health to Empower. (2015, August 13). *Carb cycling and weight loss for women.* https://www.healthtoempower.com/carb-cycling-and-weight-loss-for-women/

Hunter, G. T. (2018, August 14). *Carb cycling can boost workouts and weight loss (but there's a catch).* https://www.getthegloss.com/article/the-pros-and-cons-of-carb-cycling-for-better-workouts-and-weight-loss

Kallmyer, T. (2019, September 27). *How to calculate your macros to transform your body.* https://healthyeater.com/how-to-calculate-your-macros

Krupp, A. (2020, February 24). *Cycle syncing: Matching your health style to your menstrual cycle.* https://www.healthline.com/health/womens-health/guide-to-cycle-syncing-how-to-start#four-phases-of-cycle-syncing

Mawer, R. M. (2017, June 12). *What is carb cycling and how does it work?* https://www.healthline.com/nutrition/carb-cycling-101#section1

Natural Fit Foodie. (2019, November 8). *How to cycle sync your diet (with recipes).* https://naturalfitfoodie.com/eat-menstrual-cycle/

Ryan, D., Candeias, V., & Jorgensen, L. (2018, May 17). *We need to change the way we think about obesity.* https://www.weforum.org/agenda/2018/05/we-need-to-change-the-narrative-around-obesity-heres-why/

Sweet, J. (2018, August 3). *What is carb cycling and does it work? Here's what experts say.* https://www.healthyway.com/content/what-is-carb-cycling/